Not Just a Nurse

A Memoir and a Promise Kept

LEIGH BLACK nee CORNWELL

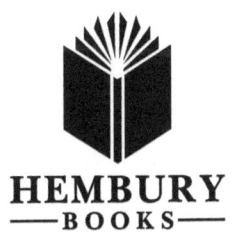

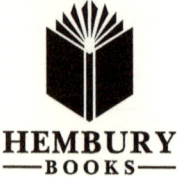

HEMBURY
—BOOKS—

Copyright © Leigh Black 2026
First published by Hembury Books in 2026
hemburybooks.com.au
info@hemburybooks.com
Paperback ISBN 9781923517639
Ebook ISBN 9781923517622

The moral right of the author has been asserted.
All rights reserved. No portion of this book may be reproduced in any form without permission from the author and publisher, except as permitted by Australian copyright law.

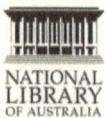 A catalogue record for this book is available from the National Library of Australia

Not Just a Nurse is dedicated to all who love, nurture and strive to make a difference

Leigh tells a tale of devotion, courage and discovery which is rich with love of her family, devotion to all her endeavours, wonder for culture and the mutual respect that comes from immersing her professional and personal skills in all that she does.

After 35 years as a GP, in both mainstream and Aboriginal community settings, I can attest that health care is complex and challenging, frustrating and fulfilling, and the best outcomes often come from relationships and connections fostered over time and sprinkled with the secret sauce of understanding and empowerment of our patients or clients.

In her own, self-deprecating though strongly determined way, Leigh's journey shows us all the potency of human connection and advocacy to truly making a difference and should inspire us all to strive for that which may at first seem unattainable.

Dr Michael Bartram, B. Med., F.R.A.C.G.P.

A beautiful retelling of stories that make up the tapestry of rural and remote nursing. Leigh brings the reader as close to the reality of rural life as possible through the written word. Respectfully telling the stories of Australia's First Nations people, Leigh gives compassionate insight into the challenges that are faced by not only Indigenous Australians, but those working with them.

In my mind's eye, I can hear the voices and see the faces of the characters she has described. This book will be enjoyed by anyone who has had the privilege of working in remote Australia, either in health or on the land.

Ruth Ni Scanlain Hackett,
Emergency Nurse Practitioner

Not Just a Nurse is a beautifully written memoir.
A story of identity, purpose and the intersections of health, culture and country.
With a love of nature, family and rural life Leigh's stories of people and places take us on the adventure of her long and active life.
Leigh's writing also captures the emotional weight of a life dedicated to service while offering insights into personal grief, systemic injustices and the cultural complexities of working, raising a family and living in rural and remote Australia.
A moving and necessary contribution to nursing literature, stories that shape our nation and Australian storytelling.

Natasha Gilmour, The Kind Press.

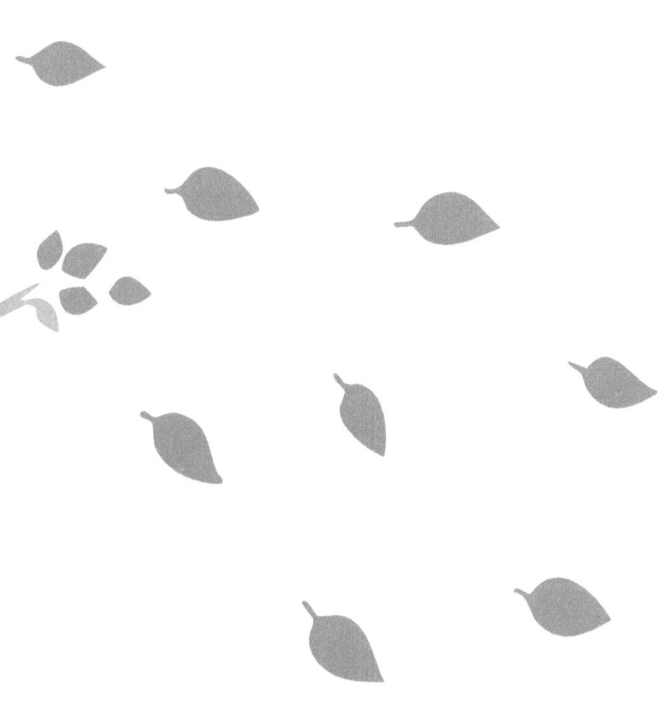

ABOUT THE AUTHOR

Leigh Black graduated as a registered nurse from Royal North Shore Hospital, Sydney, in 1973. With a career spanning 50 years, Leigh's nursing experience has been primarily in rural and remote care.

Raising children, while working in the family farming business, necessitated a hiatus from nursing. Leigh's entrepreneurial spirit was allowed some freedom though as she made a bold attempt to market Australian wool to the USA, built a successful rural tour business and during some tough years Leigh became a drought welfare officer for the Department of Primary Industries.

On returning to her primary profession in 1996, Leigh followed her dream of remote and indigenous nursing.

The experience of those years compelled Leigh to share her stories of the incredible people she met, and the wonderful places in which she was privileged to work, in her debut book *Not Just a Nurse*.

Now retired from nursing, Leigh lives in the eclectic community of Lightning Ridge, Yuwaalaraay Country, NSW where she welcomes guests to her holiday cottage on the opal fields. Time with family and friends, writing, reading and travelling are Leigh's favourite pursuits.

CONTENTS

About the author 6
Prologue 8

PART ONE
Chapter one – In their footsteps 10
Chapter two – The 'ridge 13
Chapter three – Olly and Joe 18
Chapter four – On call 22
Chapter five – Connections 24
Chapter six – Across the Nullarbor Plain 27
Chapter seven – Up north 30
Chapter eight – Joan 32
Chapter nine – Clinic hours 39
Chapter ten – Helena 48
Chapter eleven – Sandra 52

PART TWO
Chapter twelve – Ricky and Rosemary 58
Chapter thirteen – An opportunity 61
Chapter fourteen – Karratha and Mt Welcome Stations 63
Chapter fifteen – Reality 65
Chapter sixteen – A treasure chest 67
Chapter seventeen – Millie 69
Chapter eighteen – Trauma 71
Chapter nineteen – Muster season 73
Chapter twenty – Spirit world 79

PART THREE
Chapter twenty-one – Why a nurse? 89
Chapter twenty-two – Sliding doors 95
Chapter twenty-three – Family time 98
Chapter twenty-four – Grief 106
Chapter twenty-five – Self care 110
Chapter twenty-six – The 'good old days' 113

An Ethical Statement 'Not the bruises' 115
Author's notes 116
Final word 118
Acknowledgements 119
Books Mentioned 120

PROLOGUE

Ieramagadu (Roebourne), Western Australia
June 2016

It is like being in a foreign country, the gabbled, lilting sound of an ancient language, with names of people and places my tongue just cannot seem to manage.

Sometimes an experience is so vast and ongoing that it is difficult to find the words. As a result, I struggle to convey just how deeply I am touched by the stories and lives of the people I am working with and for. The horror of disadvantage and the reality of remote Aboriginal ill health is draining. Yet my spirit is buoyed by cultural connection, access to their magnificent Country, their generosity of spirit and willingness to share, their unique sense of humour, the fluency of local language and family, always family.

I am writing as a form of therapy, and I promise to one day share some of the stories. I feel compelled to do so because I know many of my friends and colleagues will never have the privilege of spending time with an Aboriginal person who was 'born on Country'. I find that sad, as there is an inherent fear of those we do not understand, and from fear grows judgement.

Aboriginal Australians are our people. Their ancestors have cared for and loved this magnificent country for more than 65,000 years. White settlement changed their lives irrevocably, and yet we know so little of their culture and language.

Lightning Ridge, New South Wales 2025

This book is my promise kept.

PART ONE

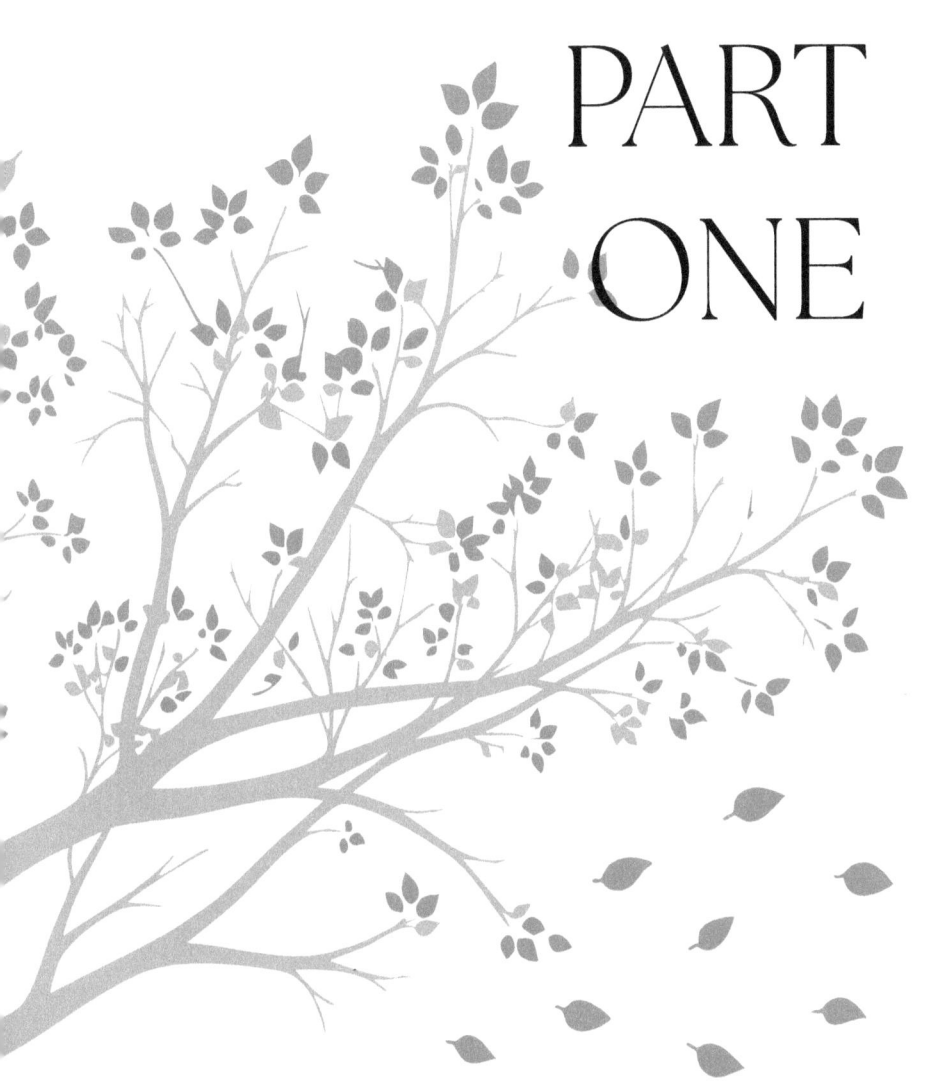

CHAPTER ONE
In their footsteps

On a bus bound for Mikra War Cemetery at Thessaloniki, in Greece, I listened to a phone message: 'Who do you think you are – you are just a nurse.'

The voice recalled to my mind a man who had not coped well with a long-past rejection. The comment made me reflective. Women of my generation have evolved past the 'not enough', 'stay quiet', 'don't stand out' mantra; however, we remain sensitive to the put-down.

It was ironic that surrounding me, on that day, were thirty-plus professional Australian and New Zealand female nurses, most coming to the last years of their working lives. All those joyous, kind, animated faces and work-worn hands. All the stories – of careers, of birth and death, of families raised, communities supported, adventures had, men and women loved – all hidden behind a cacophony of chatter.

None of us were JUST a nurse!

It was 2015. We had gathered in Athens to begin an exploration of World War I memorial graves, visit Gallipoli and to re-enact the WWI ANZAC nurses' landing on the Greek Island of Lemnos. Their task had been herculean. To establish a field hospital on a barren parcel of land, Turk's Head on the Portiano Peninsula, Lemnos. This was the closest allied-held land for those injured on Gallipoli to be evacuated to.

Cruising on the *Serenissima* from Athens to Istanbul, our small-group adventure was organised by nurse historian Dr Clare Ashton. One hundred years since the initial landing at Gallipoli in

Turkey, a series of commemorations honoured that fateful time in Australian history. An ABC series *The Anzac Girls*, inspired by the book of the same name by Peter Rees, had raised public interest in the re-enactment of the nurses' landing on Lemnos. We felt very privileged to walk in the footsteps of those brave women from one hundred years ago.

With generosity, the ABC wardrobe department had gifted the uniforms made for the series. Unfortunately, the size 8 and 10 waistbands, made to fit svelte young actresses, were no match for thickening, middle-aged waists, so much alteration was needed. Preparing and wearing my replica uniform was a very humbling experience. I felt so proud to be a nurse! I need to also add that there was shared laughter as we older nurses remembered our nursing training days, when our uniforms had changed very little from those we wore on that day.

The plan, for those doing the re-enactment, was to be taken from the *Serenissima* by tender and then to walk through the water onto the shore at Turks Head, as the nurses had one hundred years before.

At the time, tragically, many Syrian people were escaping by sea and seeking refuge on Greek and Turkish shores. Landing from the sea was deemed illegal. Instead, we berthed at Myrina Port on a day that had dawned bright with a magic sunrise, then travelled by bus ... to the most barren of landscapes. The site of what had once been a huge field hospital was bare as it had been one hundred years ago. None of us could begin to imagine the work, hardship and heartbreak that had faced those brave women in 1915.

Excitement, a feeling of reverence, expectation, reflection and sharing with fellow nurses – past and present – it was quite surreal to walk in the steps of those young women of one hundred years ago. On a 35-degree morning, walking in formation and standing through the ceremonies, those of us in uniform felt just a little of the discomfort our nurses had endured all those years ago. Just as they had, we were glad to cool off by paddling in the harbour shallows – stockings on! We did wonder how anyone survived the uniforms, both military and nursing, during WWI. Made of heavy wool or thick linen fabric, they were prickly and restrictive.

After a poignant visit to Portiano Cemetery, where far too many ANZAC soldiers and nurses are buried, we enjoyed a memorable lunch hosted by the people of Lemnos in Moudros village square. Gathered under the shade of ancient olive trees it was a welcome relief to the emotion and heat of the morning. A very real bond of shared history remains between our countries, and we were embraced just as our ancestors had been.

The emotion of the day would never be forgotten. On a ten-day memorial voyage there were also many other impactful experiences. I have so much gratitude to Dr Clare Ashton for making her dream our reality!

Our visit to the Gallipoli Peninsula in Turkey was heart-wrenching. The Turkish military base, where Florence Nightingale had laboured and is honoured, was intimidating. And then there was the service held over the site in the Aegean Sea, where the hospital ship *TS Marquette* was sunk. One of the New Zealand nurses travelling with us read pages of a diary written by her grandmother, recounting her experience of the sinking and its tragic aftermath. A simple yet compelling account from a WW1 nurse, the diary was only found in recent years, following the death of our friend's mother. The stories and the pain that was never shared.

My paternal grandfather served on Gallipoli and survived, while a maternal great-uncle was injured, taken to Lemnos, then sent on to Egypt, where he died. That young man kept a diary until two days before his death – a tragic yet wonderful personal account that remained hidden for two generations. His distraught but very religious mother had apparently kept it secret, as her nineteen-year-old son had written of his visit to an Egyptian brothel before being sent to Gallipoli.

Like many of the nurses I shared the voyage with, I was only one generation removed from the lifelong impact of those mass tragedies.

CHAPTER TWO
The 'ridge

At the time of going on that adventure, I had just completed a contract as a GP practice nurse in Pemberton, in the southwest corner of Western Australia.

My permanent home, however, was in Lightning Ridge, on Yuwaalaraay Country, New South Wales, where I had spent some years nursing.

Our daughter, Rebel, first came to Lightning Ridge as the editor of the *Ridge News*. Her dad, Rick, and I were concerned about her choice, as Rebel was only 21, and the town's mining culture, remoteness and mix of nationalities gave it a wild and eccentric reputation. On our first visit, Rebel said she would meet us at the pub as we were arriving after work on a Friday. When we arrived, I immediately felt out of place and overdressed for the local crowd. Rebel sat me opposite two men in the beer garden while Rick and Rebel pushed their way through the crowd to the bar. One of the men was a bear of a man named Ox. He leant across the table and said, 'Bet you're worried about your little girl being up here.'

'Yes, I am,' I replied quite timidly.

'Don't worry,' he said. 'I've been watching her, and she's a good girl – treats everyone the same and isn't flirtatious ... and if anyone touches her, I'll put them down a mine hole!'

'Oh, thank you, Mr Ox!' I replied.

I have loved Ox ever since.

'Mr Ox to you,' he says.

He is a man, like many in the 'ridge, with an interesting past and the older he gets, the more he likes to share his stories. Of Sicilian-Anglo heritage, he was given the title 'Ox' by the great Ron Barassi after a notable feat of strength. An early runaway, Ox tells stories of living on Maroubra Beach at thirteen, walking greyhounds for a living and becoming a volunteer lifesaver, progressing to playing rugby union for Randwick. Ox says the plumbing trade took him into the fortress home of crime boss Lenny McPherson, and he later spent years working as a doorman for Abe Saffron in nightclubs such at Les Girls, Beef and Bourbon, Chequers and Hawaiian Eye. He speaks of meeting Frank Sinatra, Tina Turner, Carlotta and describes Eartha Kitt as the most sensual woman he has ever met. A man who partied hard, Ox is not someone lesser men would mess with, and he admits to shimmying on the wrong side of the law at times.

Ox is now a much smaller version of the larger-than-life, big-muscled man he once was. When life – his big heart – finally caught up with him, I had the honour of hefting him onto a resuscitation bed and working as hard as I ever have, alongside the on-call GP, to resuscitate and stabilise him. Ultimately, we handed him over to the Royal Flying Doctor Service (RFDS) retrieval team. Ox's heart was patched, and I will always remain grateful for his life, when we stop for a yarn.

When I first came to Lightning Ridge for a six-week nursing contract in 2002, there was no hospital, just an accident and emergency unit with two resuscitation beds and two holding beds. It was open from 7 am to 10 pm and was staffed by a registered nurse, an enrolled nurse, and a security guard. Tragically, a young, registered nurse had been murdered not long before in a neighbouring town, so a security guard was deemed vital – particularly as each night one of the RNs (four on rotating shifts) was on call for any presenting emergencies.

Our regular security guard was an efficient and kind man with a quiet authority who always beat the on-call nurse to the front door to unlock for the needy patient. We were to present within seven minutes of call out under the guidelines set, no doubt, by someone who didn't have to do battle with a bra.

One night, a newly employed security guard – who had not been briefed on the seven-minute rule – walked to the site from his home. Consequently, I was in the unit alone with three young men, obviously drunk and/or drug affected, outside the door. One fellow had fallen in a fire and was screaming in pain. The glass security door did little to hide their agitation or muffle the abusive language and screams from their side. Even though the fire had been doused, I was very aware that the man's flesh would still be burning.

I recognised one of the men as an acquaintance of my opal-mining son-in-law. So, with all the authority I could muster, I unlocked the door, told them I was Mick's mother-in-law – so not to be messed with – allowed the injured man in, supported by the one I recognised and sent the other home. The new security guard arrived during the treatment phase, the on-call doctor presented, and the language and pain settled with care and tolerance. Eventually, the RFDS retrieval took place.

Quite shaken by the events of that night, and unhappy that the new security guard had not been briefed correctly, I wrote an incident report. The upshot of that was a right royal telling-off and a threatened dismissal, for me, for breaching security guidelines! The on-call doctor was a staunch ally and stated that morally, I had done the right thing by allowing the patient access to care.

With hindsight, I recognise that the manager came from her own place of fear, as it was on her watch that the young nurse had been murdered. However, it took me a while to get over my perceived injustice of the tirade I had experienced.

A funny aside to that incident was that once the patient was discharged from the base hospital, he had to regularly return to the unit for dressings, which were attended to by a young male nurse who was very protective of me. Ron told the patient how abusive he and his mate had been on that night, that I had nearly lost my job by letting him in and that he must never speak to a woman like that again.

Twenty years on, that man remains super polite to me every time he sees me.

Those same twenty years have seen me attend Ron's wedding in County Kildare, Ireland, to his Irish bride, Jennifer, who he met when they both worked at Prince of Wales Hospital in Sydney. In 2022, I made a return trip to their lovely home on the edge of the Bog of Allen, where they are raising two beautiful sons while continuing to progress their nursing careers. I know Ron keeps his Australian heritage alive with tales of his time in the 'ridge.

There is something very special about friendship across generations – friendships forged in the face of witnessing tragedy, in saving lives and in needing to rely on and support each other when there is no one else.

During Ron's employment, his mum and a friend came to visit from Victoria. Ron was anxious to show them the best of Lightning Ridge. I was happy to extend my hospitality, so while Ron was doing an evening shift, I held a small dinner party in their honour. We ladies were being well entertained by the mining adventure stories of a charming Croatian fellow when I got a call from Ron – he was going to be late off duty because a woman had presented in advanced labour. At the time, Ron was a very young man, working alongside another young male registered nurse – neither with any obstetric experience – and he sounded panicked. I offered to come to the unit … quickly … offer accepted … and the baby was safely delivered.

With adrenaline pumping, tears of relief flowed in private. I doubt either of those young men have forgotten witnessing their first birth!

The presence of a GP in town was a constant source of anxiety, a 'luck of the draw' situation when it came to their experience and first line emergency skills. Those years before a hospital was built were hectic, adrenaline-packed and at times frightening, as our presentations ranged from the need for a pair of crutches to a full-scale trauma.

I, and others, were not fully equipped to deal with so many of the presentations. However, we did – we had no choice. We drew on each other's skill base, those of the ambulance officers, the ever-present security person, basic first-line care, common sense and compassion.

The extraordinary service of the Royal Flying Doctor Service was, and remains, a godsend, with their retrieval service called on a regular basis. Our RFDS centre is now in Dubbo, which is a four-hour drive by road ambulance. During my first years working in Lightning Ridge, we were linked to Broken Hill RFDS, and it was to their doctors that a registered nurse would speak if no local GP was available. Broken Hill is located on the far western border of New South Wales, is much closer to Adelaide, the capital city of South Australia, than to Dubbo or Sydney. The distances are vast, across flat, arid country and the resources small.

I was at a conference some years ago where we were all asked to stand, introduce ourselves and state where we currently worked. At the next tea break, a RFDS doctor bounded up to me, arms outstretched in greeting – we had shared a very tense night. I had been in Lightning Ridge Accident and Emergency (A&E) with a patient requiring significant pain relief and no GP to order medication, while he had been inflight to Adelaide, resuscitating a critically ill patient. His terse order to 'give the patient whatever you think necessary' was a huge risk for both of us, but it was also a sign of the working trust that a remote emergency situation calls for. I was told at one stage by management that NSW Health would cover us in those situations. Despite requesting, I never did get that in writing!

The education and employment of nurse practitioners is a practical solution to many similar scenarios.

There is a plethora of stories from that time, some too traumatic to articulate, and in respect of confidentiality, not suitable to disclose. However, others are recalled easily, particularly those involving two colleagues who taught me so much during my first months in the 'ridge.

CHAPTER THREE
Olly and Joe

My first Christmas on duty was only six weeks after I had left the security of my dearly loved rural home. The morning, on my own, was very challenging as I reflected on the many years of noisy, wonderful family Christmases. At the height of menopause, in the middle of a drought cycle, and adjusting to an empty nest, my husband's decision to sell our family home and property had led to a pending divorce, a shared staff rental home and distance from friends, family and animals ... all weighed heavily.

However, I had a job to do, as I was on an afternoon/evening shift.

Joe, my colleague, had just left the building after a quiet morning shift when the phone rang. The ambulance service gave warning that a major, single-person trauma was about to present. I called Joe back! That shift became an ongoing nightmare as other patients came and went, some were treated, while others just went home realising that they weren't in desperate need.

All the while, efforts to stabilise a severely battered young body continued, as arrangements were made for his air retrieval by the Royal Flying Doctor Service critical care team to an intensive care unit.

I recall Joe and me sharing the clean-up after the retrieval ... literally mopping up blood and other fluids at 2 am.

'Merry Christmas, eh?' says Joe – master of the understatement.

I needed to catch a couple of hours sleep as I was to be back in the unit at 7 am.

Boxing Day was known to be a very busy one. Strangely, there were always a lot of vomiting bugs around (nothing to do with overindulgence, of course) and there was an extra registered nurse sharing the shift.

I had been told the RN, Olly, came from Wanaaring and was visiting family in the 'ridge. 'Oh golly, its Olly' – known for her radio call and as Australia's very first remote nurse practitioner. Her reputation preceded her. I was in awe, and I was very nervous!

My years of nursing have spanned from the crisp veil, rigidly starched full aprons, thick brown stockings and serious fully enclosed leather shoes to scrubs and joggers, however at this time, our Area Health Service had embraced the 'corporate uniform'. Dutifully, I made sure mine was well-pressed and clean prior to bed that morning, adding my blazer for good measure. I was to work in such illustrious company. To be honest, the adrenaline was still pumping, so little sleep was had!

Olly arrived, late, sporting spiked, pink-dyed, cropped hair, a pair of trackie dacks and an oversized T-shirt. That woman was a statement in joggers.

We got to work. One of our first presentations was a young female overdosing on a substance unknown. Using all my best words for drug choices while questioning her friends, I got my first lesson from Olly. The girl was deteriorating, her friends were not giving any information, it was getting tense. Olly knew the boyfriend and took over questioning, impressively using all the street names for possible drugs ingested, but the response remained silence and shifting eyes. Until Olly grabbed the boy by his shirt, pushed him against the wall, looked him in the eye and said, 'If you don't fucking tell me what she's taken, she will die, and I will kill you!' Yes, unorthodox, but it worked. He talked, the girl got the treatment she needed, and I quickly adopted the local vernacular for street drugs.

Late morning, there was a break in the patient load, and we took the opportunity to grab a coffee and sit outside. Olly gave me a quizzical look and asked what my story was. I stammered something about grown kids and pending divorce, to which she said, 'Oh, you'll be looking for a bloke then.'

I stated that it was not on my mind at present, and she replied, 'Well, you tell me when you start looking, because in this town you can get two things from a bloke – an STD or an opal – you tell me who you are looking at and I will tell you what you will get.'

Ever direct was Olly!

Olly took a position at Goodooga, a small Indigenous community 70 odd kilometres north-west of Lightning Ridge, so she could be closer to her family, and we became firm friends. I credit her for teaching me, by example, what it was to truly be a remote nurse. I remember going to functions with Olly, she would inevitably end up with mothers and babes yarning about whether the kids were vaccinated or talking to some old fellow who hadn't turned up for a treatment.

Olly lost her own health battle far too young. I had a poem which we both loved. On the evening of International Women's Day, I was part of a large gathering of women under a wonderful starry, western sky. We were sharing poetry, and I preceded my reading of *After a While* by Veronica A. Shoffstall by saying Olly was very ill in Sydney and I was dedicating the poem to her. About five minutes after I finished reciting, my phone rang. Olly had passed. I like to think she left this world with the collective love of her female community giving her wings.

My colleague Joe was one of the first male registered nurses and had trained in Townsville, Queensland. If Joe was on duty everyone felt safe, he had been in the 'ridge for years. He had seen it all.

I, on the other hand, seemed to have come from another planet and I had the ability to say really dumb things in his company. One Sunday, I came to work and to make conversation, as you do when your colleague probably wishes you wouldn't, I said I had taken rubbish to the tip that morning.

'Been a lot of money made from that hole,' Joe said.

'Oh Joe, there isn't that much money in scrap metal, is there?' I replied.

Joe lowered his glasses and looked at me. 'This is an opal mining town, Leigh.'

Duh!

We experienced some very hectic shifts over that first Christmas and New Year period. As Joe went off shift on New

Year's Eve, he suggested I come to the club after I finished at 10 pm – we deserved a drink.

I then asked him if he would please meet me outside when I got there.

'Why?'

I told him I had never walked into a place like that on my own, I had been married for twenty-eight years.

With no pity he said, 'Get over it!'

I took a deep breath, and I did. Walked all the way through the mostly intoxicated crowd to the bar, where Joe greeted me with a Sambuca. Never had one of those before either! I was on the road to confident independence.

Joe has a very dry humour which was not often evident in the workplace. One afternoon, we had a 'love triangle' arrive by ambulance, with police close behind. The threesome were off their faces and both men were covered in a lot of blood from multiple knife wounds. The new boyfriend had an arterial wound at his elbow that was literally pumping blood. While the ambulance officers and police looked after the more superficially injured ex-boyfriend, Joe and I got to work on the arterial wound. Couldn't get rid of the girlfriend, though. As we worked, she straddled the poor bloke and sexily massaged his chest with his own blood. I don't want to know where her head was, but at least it kept her quiet and non-violent. It was bizarre.

The tension of stabilising the patient was broken when, out of the blue, Joe said, 'Ain't love grand?'

Incidentally, at the point of the patient's retrieval, we realised by a chance remark that the woman was the perpetrator!

CHAPTER FOUR
On call

I remember one horrible, all-night ordeal.
A call-out about midnight for an ambulance admission carrying a male patient with a suspected head injury. Following a very vague history handover, the male ambulance officers left. Then, the patient's behaviour escalated to extreme verbal abuse and non-compliance – he simply would not allow me to examine him. The security man could do little; in fact, his presence seemed to distress the patient more. The on-call male doctor was tired and intolerant of the man's behaviour and left me to do 'whatever you think needs to be done.'

In my rush to get to the unit that night, I had slipped on a T-shirt clearly labelled with '*Practice Nurses Association*'. At one stage, the fellow screamed at me 'What the fuck is a practice nurse doing here anyway. You aren't even qualified!'

I wondered the same. At least I knew the fellow's eyesight was not impaired by his head injury.

Policing in Lightning Ridge was limited and even by the standards of the time, appalling. Multiple calls for support saw one policeman arrive at about 3.30 am. On hearing the tirade of abuse and witnessing the patient's behaviour he stated 'This doesn't look good. I had better go home and get my belt on.'

Then he left.

I am not sure how far away home was, but I was subjected to another ninety minutes of threats, if I approached the patient, along with ongoing verbal abuse. Two police officers finally arrived, belts equipped with a gun, handcuffs and assorted implements, fastened around their waists.

An arrest took place. The patient was escorted from the unit. I was relieved but also distressed. Other than a patient being removed in a body bag, there is no worse feeling for someone trained to care for those in crisis than to see a patient leave in handcuffs.

I went home as dawn was breaking. I wasn't due back in the unit until 2 pm, so I poured a glass of wine, lit a cigarette, sat on my verandah and cried. I recall saying out loud, 'This town will ruin me!'

Smoking and drinking were strictly an after dark special occasion treat in my normal life. However, this was far from my normal.

While working that afternoon, a senior ambulance officer called in to check on my wellbeing which I greatly appreciated. Being the subject of someone's ranting abuse for hours on end is not pleasant and I was shaken. I was also very curious – why? The Ambo informed me that word on the street was that our patient had done a bad drug deal and his life was at risk. His only way out of town safely, therefore, was in police custody. So, he had contrived an accident with head injury, behaved very badly in care and got himself arrested.

There are times I hope karma is a thing.

On leaving my position, which had transitioned into a 24-hour care Multipurpose Service (MPS), after five years, I remember thanking the universe that my patients and I had survived my lack of formal intensive care, midwifery, trauma, mental health and cardiac training.

Bizarrely, the first day I walked into that unit, I suddenly recalled walking past it many years before while on a weekend away with my young husband and our babies. I remember thinking, *I would love to work there one day.*

I had not thought of it since.

Be careful what you wish for as the universe hears!

CHAPTER FIVE
Connections

One of the many GPs who rotated through the Lightning Ridge A&E for two weeks was a delightful gentleman from New Zealand named Dr Tripe. He never returned to the 'ridge, however my dear mother, who lived in our hometown of Coonabarabran, started speaking of Dr Tripe who was accepting regular locum contracts in that town and had become a firm favourite of Mum's. I was staying with Mum when Dr Tripe made an unexpected house call, and he immediately recognised me. He asked me what I was doing there. Apparently, he remembered me as being professionally effective during an emergency we were both involved with.

It possibly says more about the ongoing trauma I had worked in that I did not remember the incident. He swore that because of it, he would never work in a remote and professionally unsupported location again.

This conversation and reconnection was of course music to my proud mother's ears.

Mum, Gwen, was a very sociable lady and when, during the conversation, it was disclosed that Dr Tripe had his wife with him during his stay in Coonabarabran, Mum asked her to afternoon tea.

Dr Clare Ashton, Nurse Historian, enjoyed afternoon tea with my mother and during the ensuing conversation, Clare told Mum about her plans for the re-enactment of the nurses' landing on Lemnos.

Mum decreed that I would do that trip, and there was no arguing with my mother.

Aside from the wonder of travel, the conversations enjoyed, and extraordinary experiences gained, there were two direct outcomes from that journey my mother said that I would take. Mum insisted on paying for my adventure. I am fiercely independent and felt I could meet the cost myself, so I argued the point. Mum bluntly told me, 'Leigh, you will inherit some money from me so by taking some now, at least I can enjoy watching you spend it.' By arguing I realised I was taking pleasure from Mum, who had been unable to give me very much as a child and was now able to do so. Humbled, I accepted graciously!

A feeling of obligation then ensured that I kept a comprehensive diary of the journey and took many photos to share with Mum on my return. Records to be treasured.

I have now passed on to my own children the promised gift of a shared travel experience to be taken in their forties, so I am not too old to share it. To date, Rebel, my eldest, and I have shared two weeks of trekking in Nepal, which was an extraordinary experience and is a heartfelt memory.

The second outcome was professional.

I had fallen in love with a man in Pemberton, WA, which was wonderful, however I felt my career was petering out into something I no longer had a heart for. After working in remote and rather tough locations, I found being a practice nurse to the lovely people of Pemberton, with their first world illnesses, professionally rather boring if I am to be honest. I had a very strong feeling that I had wasted the potential of my nursing career and that my skill base was not grounded in science as I had not sought academic achievement.

Nearing retirement, I was a jack of all trades, full of self-doubt and disappointment in my career choices.

And then the cruise happened.

I remained very quiet amongst some highly qualified academic nurses. For days, I felt quite intimidated by the achievements that some of those urban-living women spoke of.

Eventually though, the story of how I met Dr Tripe was spoken of, my rural and remote location became known, and I was treated with a respect that shocked me. These wonderful professional women thought what I had done with my life and career was amazing and brave.

We all have a role. My confidence was boosted as I started to recognise my own skills, which were based not on science or academic achievement but in advocacy, compassion, practical care and a lived understanding of the environment that my patients came from.

CHAPTER SIX
Across the Nullarbor Plain

The Royal Flying Doctor Service relies heavily on the Australian public for donations to maintain its service. In 2011, a group of retired friends from Mudgee – cycling enthusiasts, entertainers and intrepid campers – decided to cycle from Darwin to Broome, fundraising for the RFDS along the way.

Great idea.

Of course I would join them!

But first, I needed to buy a bike and learn to ride it. Horses had always been my preferred mode of leisure and work transport. That trip, as an older inexperienced rider, was singularly the most stupid thing I have ever done but what an adventure it was. The team rode 1,800 kilometres, averaging 100 kilometres per day, and we raised $28,000 dollars along the way.

That extraordinary adventure reignited an old dream of mine – to work in Indigenous health in the Kimberley region. In 2013, I returned to Darwin for a dream holiday cruising down the Kimberley coast to Broome.

The north of Western Australia had captured my heart.

My beloved stepfather and father-in-law died as dignified elder men within six months of my 60th birthday. Both were WWII veterans who had led honourable and loving lives. My first precious grandchild had been born; my children were established and happy in their lives and my dear mother was supported by family and friends and was still independent.

I was restless.

Rural Health West (RHW) is a medical recruitment agency in Western Australia. It was RHW that organised my position in Pemberton in the southwest of Western Australia, which was for a five-month contract. RHW recruiting staff were aware that I had wanted to work in the Kimberley, however only year-long contracts could be offered. I felt that I couldn't leave my family or home for a year, so I accepted the Pemberton role – based on the knowledge that it was close to Margaret River, well known for its fine wine production and scenic coastline.

My family were gracious, my friends encouraging and a young colleague offered to stay in my home and take care of my lovely Labrador dog Millie. There was only fear of change and loneliness to overcome. With car laden, my kayak on the roof and that bike on the back, I set off to drive across Australia – 3,800 kilometres from Lightning Ridge to Pemberton, Western Australia. It was a grand adventure. The stirring music of Queen rocked me across the iconic Nullarbor Plain. I didn't rush the journey as this was a special time of freedom for me, and I was only to be away for five months.

My final day's drive to Pemberton from Albany via Denmark and Northcliffe was intimidating. The majestic karri forests of the region towered over me. The narrow, winding roads and stormy skies added to a feeling of gloom and peril. I was used to vast plains and blue skies. I was grateful that my morning coffee had been shared with two Indigenous women who welcomed me to their Country and told me of the delightful taste of Marron which is native to the waterways of that fertile area of Western Australia. The welcome to my new home, after such a drive, was a wonderful homemade pasta and red wine-fuelled dinner party hosted by my new house mate, an Italian trainee GP named Roberta. So many years my junior, we were both far from home and quickly developed a heartfelt relationship that has been a delight to me over the years.

Pemberton is a place of abundance, rich in agricultural and logging history and pioneered by both Italian and English families. In living memory, the undulating rich-soil country was cleared of its mighty trees. Generational wealth was made by hard labour and the planting of potatoes, grapes, fruit trees and pasture for cattle.

While adjusting to such a different landscape, I often walked to the main town oval just to get a sense of space. Particularly through the winter rains, there is a reason for all that green and the rainfall was a shock to my desert-country soul.

My kayak was put to good use in time, but the bike was well parked – have you seen the hills in Pemberton? I would have been terrified going down them if I ever thought it possible, for me, to peddle up them.

I settled into work in Pemberton determined to enjoy my five months, little knowing that I would only come home for holidays, the birth of grandchildren and my mum's advancing age for the next six years. I would drive across the Nullarbor Plain five more times and fly across many more.

The power of a man who, coincidentally, made his own red wine, knew the best places to catch Marron and spent his spare time fishing and boating from a rustic hut close to the river mouth of the Donnelly River – a remote and pristine paradise.

Andrew, though, is another story.

CHAPTER SEVEN
Up north

On return from the ANZAC journey, with renewed confidence and a zest for more, I spoke with Rural Health West and was subsequently alerted to two positions with a one-year contract.

One in Broome in the Kimberley, which had been my goal, as a GP practice nurse. The other as the chronic disease nurse, for an Aboriginal Medical Service, at Roebourne in the Pilbara. So, a decision… a relatively easy job in a multicultural and quite exotic tourist town or a tough job in a town I knew nothing about but was quickly told had a troubled Indigenous history?

My gut told me the hard one, so that's what I chose.

It was a long week as I said no to the Broome offer before I was even interviewed for the Roebourne position.

A leap of faith!

My heart was captured early by the people of the Pilbara and their vast, dramatic landscape. That iron-red dirt does get into your veins as well as ingraining itself in your skin and every item of clothing you own.

On the lands of the Ngarluma and Yindjibarndi people is the township of Ieramagadu (Roebourne), where people from different language groups were forced to come when they were dispossessed of their *Ngurra* (Country). Roebourne holds a special place in Indigenous cultural history as being the beginning place of the lyrical and wonderous story of the *Songline of the Seven Sisters*.

A couple of years later, at my CEO's suggestion, Andrew and I, during a trip east to family, detoured to Canberra for the exhibition

Songlines: Tracking the Seven Sisters at the National Museum of Australia. A wonderous display of art and culture and an ancient story linking the waterholes and landmarks of the desert lands from Roebourne to Uluru. Imagery and story being the ancient Indigenous way of recording and memorising Country.

In our European history, Roebourne was the first town in the state's northwest and is on the banks of the beautiful Ngurin (Harding) River, which flows out to sea at Cossack. It is close to the mining town of Wickham, the seaside community of Point Samson and 70 kilometres from the city of Karratha. There is vast wealth and privilege in the Pilbara, despite its isolation, but not in Roebourne.

The complexity of disease, social structures and overwhelming need impacts the most stoic of health practitioners when first faced with the onslaught of chronic disease in the Indigenous communities of Australia's northwest. I was so bloody shocked at the statistics that I had access to from the very well-managed database at Mawarnkarra Health Service. Screening and diagnosis are one of the great strengths of this wonderful organisation.

The chronic disease database noted 800-plus patients with more than one chronic disease. Very few were medication-compliant, many resistant to care and for most, English was their second or third language. In our first world lives, we spend time working on acceptance. However, these spiritual, culturally connected people had it in spades – but it was working against them.

It is not acceptable to be sick and dying young of diseases that the first world considers preventable and treatable, especially when living in one of the most resource-rich areas of the world. The Pilbara is these people's Country. They are culturally, physically and spiritually aligned to their place.

Surely, we can do better!

CHAPTER EIGHT
Joan

I wish to acknowledge the CEO of Mawarnkarra Health Service (MHS).

Joan Hicks is a proud Ngarluma and Yindjibarndi woman, who has raised her family in Roebourne with her partner John, a proud Yindjibarndi man.

Joan and John are an unassuming couple with a love of family, animals and country music. Joan has a gentle and quiet manner, yet she has a powerful presence. It took months before I felt she had developed any trust in my integrity.

I was relieved when John finally responded to a recall letter. As is the custom in many First Nation families, the couple do not share the same surname, so I had not made the connection until John sat down and stated that his boss and mine had told him he had to come in to see me.

Two years into my employment at Mawarnkarra, Joan's daughter came to my office. She explained that her mother's pet billy goat had become very aggressive, was charging people and had become dangerous. The family wondered if my partner, Andrew, by then Karratha and Mt Welcome Station manager, could castrate the goat. I duly asked Andrew, and he was happy to oblige. With the assistance of two young stockmen to wrestle the goat to the ground, Andrew operated. I can't imagine it was an easy job, as an adult billy goat is rather well-endowed, but all were experienced with the castrating of young bulls.

'All good,' was the report.

But not so.

I arrived at work the next morning to be sent a message that Joan's goat was dead.

OMG.

Obviously from shock, but how to face an upset Joan?

Andrew went into dramatic Italian crisis mode and was convinced he would be the cause of my dismissal.

'Sorry for your loss, Joan,' was as far as the inevitable conversation went, and the billy goat saga was never spoken of ... until discussing this writing, when Joan said, 'What about the billy goat?'

A forgiving woman.

Joan is an observer, which, to an extrovert like me, can strike fear in my heart. Typically, both personality traits align completely with our very different cultural backgrounds. We white fellas talk too much, and one of my greatest challenges in life has been to stop and listen.

In the words of Dr Miriam-Rose Ungunmerr-Baumann AM, a respected Ngan'gityemerri Elder, artist, teacher and 2021 Senior Australian of the Year.

Dadirri - A Reflection by Miriam-Rose Ungunmerr-Baumann

NGANGIKURUNGKURR means 'Deep Water Sounds'. *Ngangikurungkurr* is the name of my tribe. The word can be broken up into three parts: *Ngangi* means word or sound, *Kuri* means water, and *kurr* means deep. So the name of my people means 'the Deep Water Sounds' or 'Sounds of the Deep'. This talk is about tapping into that deep spring that is within us.

Many Australians understand that Aboriginal people have a special respect for Nature. The identity we have with the land is sacred and unique. Many people are beginning to understand this more. Also there are many Australians who appreciate that Aboriginal people have a very strong sense of community. All persons matter. All of us belong. And there are many more Australians now, who understand that we are a people who celebrate together.

What I want to talk about is another special quality of my people. I believe it is the most important. It is our most unique gift. It is perhaps the greatest gift we can give to our fellow Australians. In our language this quality is called *dadirri*. It is inner, deep listening and quiet, still awareness.

Dadirri recognises the deep spring that is inside us. We call on it and it calls to us. This is the gift that Australia is thirsting for. It is something like what you call "contemplation".

When I experience *dadirri*, I am made whole again. I can sit on the riverbank or walk through the trees; even if someone close to me has passed away, I can find my peace in this silent awareness. There is no need of words. A big part of *dadirri* is listening. Through the years, we have listened to our stories. They are told and sung, over and over, as the seasons go by. Today we still gather around the campfires and together we hear the sacred stories.

As we grow older, we ourselves become the storytellers. We pass on to the young ones all they must know. The stories and songs sink quietly into our minds and we hold them deep inside. In the ceremonies we celebrate the awareness of our lives as sacred.

The contemplative way of *dadirri* spreads over our whole life. It renews us and brings us peace. It makes us feel whole again...

In our Aboriginal way, we learnt to listen from our earliest days. We could not live good and useful lives unless we listened. This was the normal way for us to learn - not by asking questions. We learnt by watching and listening, waiting and then acting. Our people have passed on this way of listening for over 40,000 years...

There is no need to reflect too much and to do a lot of thinking. It is just being aware. My people are not threatened by silence. They are completely at home in it. They have lived for thousands of years with Nature's quietness. My people today, recognise and experience in this quietness, the great Life-Giving Spirit, the Father of us all. It is easy for me to experience God's presence. When I am out hunting, when I am in the bush, among the trees, on a hill or by a billabong; these are the times when I can simply be in God's presence. My people have been so aware of Nature. It is natural that we will feel close to the Creator.

Dr Stanner, the anthropologist who did much of his work among the Daly River tribes, wrote this: "Aboriginal religion was probably one of the least material minded, and most life-minded of any of which we have knowledge."

And now I would like to talk about the other part of *dadirri* which is the quiet stillness and the waiting.

Our Aboriginal culture has taught us to be still and to wait. We do not try to hurry things up. We let them follow their natural course - like the seasons. We watch the moon in each of its phases. We wait for the rain to fill our rivers and water the thirsty earth...

When twilight comes, we prepare for the night. At dawn we rise with the sun.

We watch the bush foods and wait for them to ripen before we gather them. We wait for our young people as they grow, stage by stage, through their initiation ceremonies.

When a relation dies, we wait a long time with the sorrow. We own our grief and allow it to heal slowly.

We wait for the right time for our ceremonies and our meetings. The right people must be present. Everything must be done in the proper way. Careful preparations must be made. We don't mind waiting, because we want things to be done with care. Sometimes many hours will be spent on painting the body before an important ceremony.

We don't like to hurry. There is nothing more important than what we are attending to. There is nothing more urgent that we must hurry away for.

We wait on God, too. His time is the right time. We wait for him to make his Word clear to us. We don't worry. We know that in time and in the spirit of *dadirri* (that deep listening and quiet stillness) his way will be clear.

We are River people. We cannot hurry the river. We have to move with its current and understand its ways.

We hope that the people of Australia will wait. Not so much waiting for us - to catch up - but waiting with us, as we find our pace in this world.

There is much pain and struggle as we wait. The Holy Father understood this patient struggle when he said to us:

"If you stay closely united, you are like a tree, standing in the middle of a bush fire sweeping through the timber. The leaves are scorched and the tough bark is scarred and burnt; but inside the tree the sap is still flowing, and under the ground the roots are still strong.

Like that tree, you have endured the flames, and you still have the power to be reborn".

My people are used to the struggle, and the long waiting. We still wait for the white people to understand us better. We ourselves had to spend many years learning about the white man's ways. Some of the learning was forced; but in many cases people tried hard over a long time, to learn the new ways.

We have learned to speak the white man's language. We have listened to what he had to say. This learning and listening should go both ways. We would like people in Australia to take time to listen to us. We are hoping people will come closer. We keep on longing for the things that we have always hoped for - respect and understanding...

To be still brings peace - and it brings understanding. When we are really still in the bush, we concentrate. We are aware of the anthills and the turtles and the water lilies.

Our culture is different. We are asking our fellow Australians to take time to know us; to be still and to listen to us...

Life is very hard for many of my people. Good and bad things came with the years of contact - and with the years following. People often absorbed the bad things and not the good. It was easier to do the bad things than to try a bit harder to achieve what we really hoped for...

I would like to conclude ... by saying again that there are deep springs within each of us.

Within this deep spring, which is the very Spirit of God, is a sound. The sound of Deep calling to Deep. The sound is the word of God - Jesus.

Today, I am beginning to hear the Gospel at the very level of my identity. I am beginning to feel the great need we have of Jesus - to protect and strengthen our identity; and to make us whole and new again.

"The time for re-birth is now," said the Holy Father to us. Jesus comes to fulfil, not to destroy.

If our culture is alive and strong and respected, it will grow. It will not die.

And our spirit will not die.

And I believe that the spirit of *dadirri* that we have to offer will blossom and grow, not just within ourselves, but in our whole nation.

When I trained as a nurse there was a very strong ethos around authority, hierarchy and discipline. We were actively taught to translate doctors' orders in plain language. Being an often falsely confident person, I embraced this role with passion as a nurse and health advocate. I can still launch into a one-sided dialogue, using appropriately simple analogies and non-medical language, which will leave the receiver with glazed eyes.

Nursing is a humbling experience, and we learn as much from our patients as they do from us. Never more so than at the end of my nursing journey at Mawarnkarra.

With no formal education, Joan started her working life in Aboriginal health as a trainee Aboriginal Health Worker in 1990. At the time, Mawarnkarra Health Service Aboriginal Corporation operated out of a house that had been converted into single men's quarters.

Over the years, Joan has worked full-time in a complex and demanding environment, raised her family, studied and risen to the top of an organisation that now oversees an astonishing range of medical, emotional, environmental and wellbeing services. If the community has need, MHS is at the forefront of service provision.

I highly recommend reading *Wandering with Intent* by Kim Mahood (published in 2022), there are so many truths in this powerful collection of essays. One paragraph struck me regarding the wisdom of Mawarnkarra Health Service as an employer:

"It is mandatory for anyone wishing to work in Antarctica to undergo a physical and psychological assessment to establish whether they will stand up to the stresses of isolation, the extreme environment and the intense proximity to other people. All the same factors exist in remote Aboriginal communities, along with confronting cross cultural conditions. Yet there don't appear to be any recognised training programs for people who aspire to work in a community, or any screening criteria to weed out the mad, bad and incompetent who prowl the grey zone of Indigenous service delivery"

Mawarnkarra not only conducts the mandatory interview and professional check process but also provides active, compulsory cultural education and weekly professional development. With the acknowledgement that staff have access to a city and airport, there is also a low tolerance for poor behaviour and a strong understanding of the personal needs of staff members. No organisation is without flaws, however, the fact that this large organisation, with its complexity of personalities and politics, functions at such a high level is testament to Joan's leadership.

The name Mawarnkarra comes from the Yindjibarndi language. Its meaning translates to 'one with power to heal', and it is pronounced *Mawarnkadda* – unless you can roll your r's really well.

Mawarnkarra Health Service is an inclusive and generous workplace.

CHAPTER NINE
Clinic hours

I have a kaleidoscope of rich and heartwarming memories of Mawarnkarra.

There is nothing more heartfelt or hectic than a clinic room filled with little people climbing over every available piece of furniture while a grandmother sits in consultation. All speaking in language, it seems at once, as I understand not one word. One quiet child, though, sits on her lap. Culturally, she is her grandmother's 'Aunty' and is learning how to care for her Grandmother as she approaches her elder years.

A routine antipsychotic injection, which any of the nurses or Aboriginal Health Workers (AHWs) could have given, was booked beside my name by request of the patient. I didn't recognise the name and was busy with a lengthy chronic disease consultation. Reception staff stated the patient would wait for me. While waiting, his family became agitated and verbal with him. Despite that, and the offer of another staff member, he waited patiently for me.

When I eventually called the patient, I was presented with a very unkept, elderly Indigenous man. His shirt was open, the scars from manhood initiation were evident. As culturally appropriate, he made no eye contact and seemed nonverbal. I was very aware that English was a third language for many of our patients. During my care of him, I asked if he could understand my English. He nodded. Toward the end of the care, I thanked him for waiting so long and asked why he had wanted to see me. Looking me straight in the eye for the first time, he said, 'I just wanted to see someone old.'

Word had spread.

God love the man. He became a regular patient of mine, and over time, our team managed to get him support for regular showers, meals and changes of clothing.

One of our patients, a man struggling with alcohol addiction, presented sober and very upset. Despite having been sober for three days, he had been denied service from the Wickham liquor outlet for being drunk. Strict liquor sale restrictions are in place at Roebourne, so our patient had made a real effort – remaining sober, cleaning up and hitchhiking to and from Wickham, a 25-kilometre round trip from his home in Roebourne. The man was understandably unhappy and requested that a doctor write a letter stating that he was sober. His plan was to take the letter back to the liquor store so he could then purchase the drinks he and his wife enjoy so much. I calmed him by saying that he was probably judged as drunk because of the way he walked, and I agreed that it was unfair to be judged that way.

As was our practice, I attended a health check and took bloods for pathology, noting ataxia – a lack of coordination, often a symptom of alcohol abuse – before the patient saw the GP doctor for his requested letter. A couple of days later, the GP came to me with the pathology results. The man had extreme magnesium deficiency, not ataxia, despite being provided with magnesium daily in his Webster pack. It was clear he hadn't been taking his medications.

I then found myself in the rather bizarre position of finding the patient to explain that if he took his tablets, his muscles would work better. Then, he wouldn't walk as if he was drunk and would be able to buy alcohol.

Country, place and family meant so much to the people that, by way of connection, I would introduce myself to a new patient by touching my opal earrings and telling patients that these gemstones represented where I came from.

One regular patient always wore the same shirt, featuring a full face of a lion. A Vinnies shirt from a long-ago Perth Zoo promotion, it had seen better days. A *lion of a man* himself, with great presence and charisma, he was now in his sixties, living with his elderly mother. A stockman for most of his life, years of hard labour and alcohol abuse was catching up with his health. I had a friend with contacts at Western Plains Zoo in Dubbo, in the northwest of NSW. I was able to get him a new lion shirt.

When I told him it was from my Country, near where my mum lived, he said, 'Please thank your mother for lending you to us.'

It reminded me of a distressing time when I had left Coonabarabran, the community where I had gone to school and had raised my children.

With great regret, I told an Indigenous woman I had worked with that I was leaving.

She said, 'The next place needs you more now.'

A profoundly comforting and freeing way of thinking.

There are so many stories.

With their permission, I wish to share just a few of the people who, to this day, remain in my thoughts and in my heart.

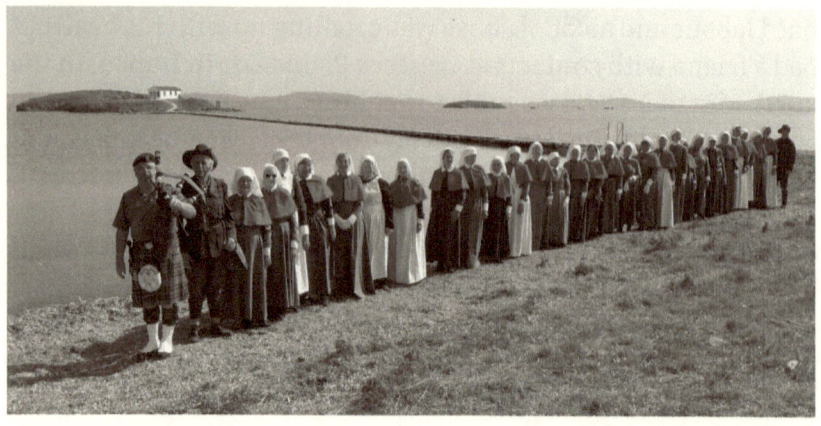

Re-enactment of the nurses landing on Lemnos Greece 2015

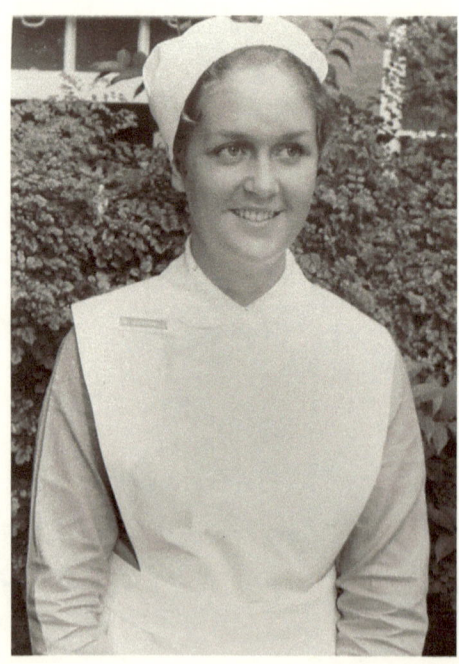

At the beginning of my nursing career Royal North Shore Hospital Sydney 1970

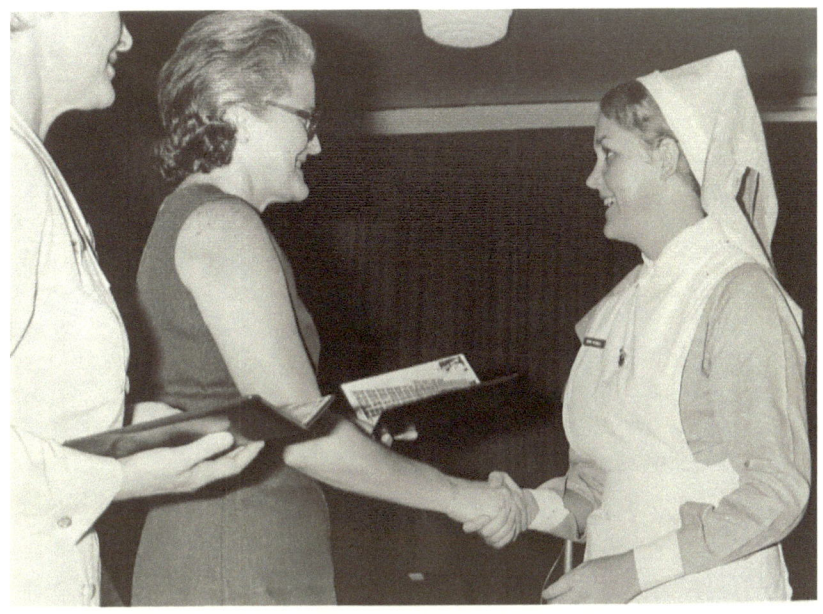

Graduation Day Royal North Shore Hospital Sydney March 1973

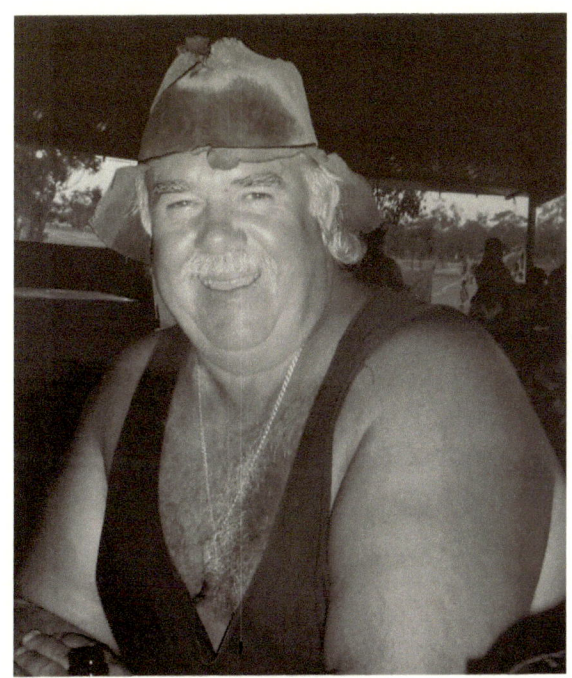

Ox back in the day
Lightning Ridge
NSW 2006

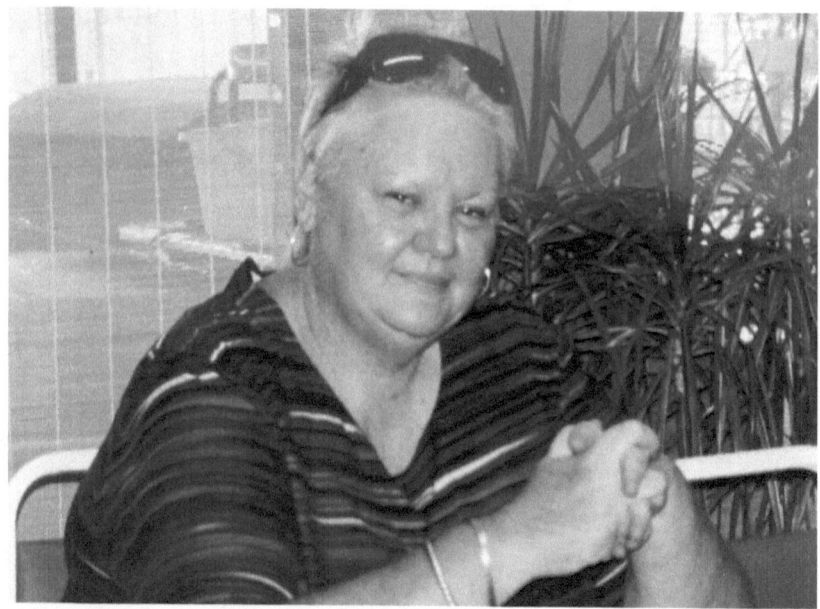

My friend and colleague Olwyn Johnson (Olly) Nurse Practitioner Lightning Ridge 2007

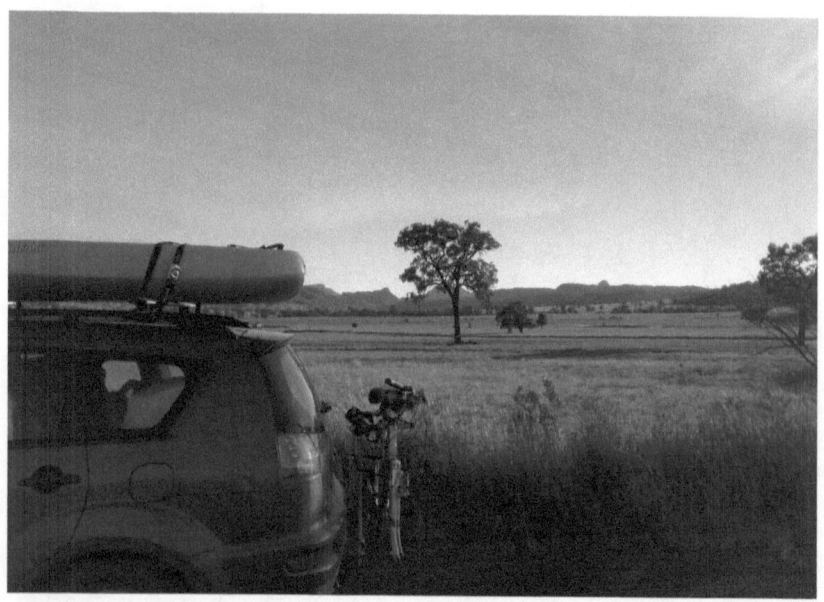

Leaving the Warrumbungle Range to drive across the Nullarbor Plain 2014

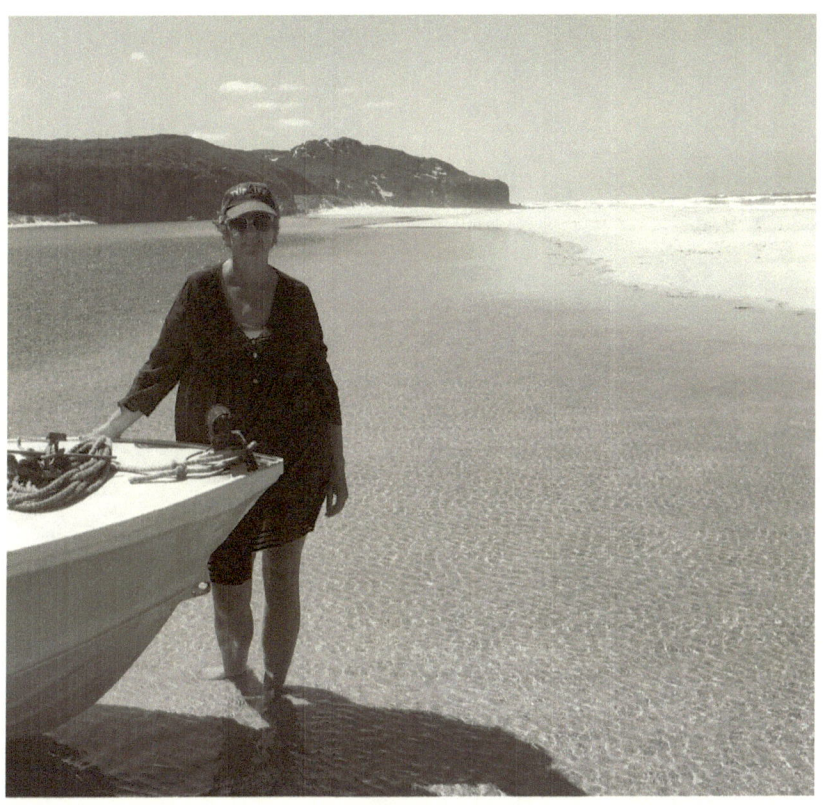

At the mouth of the Donnelly River Southwest WA 2014

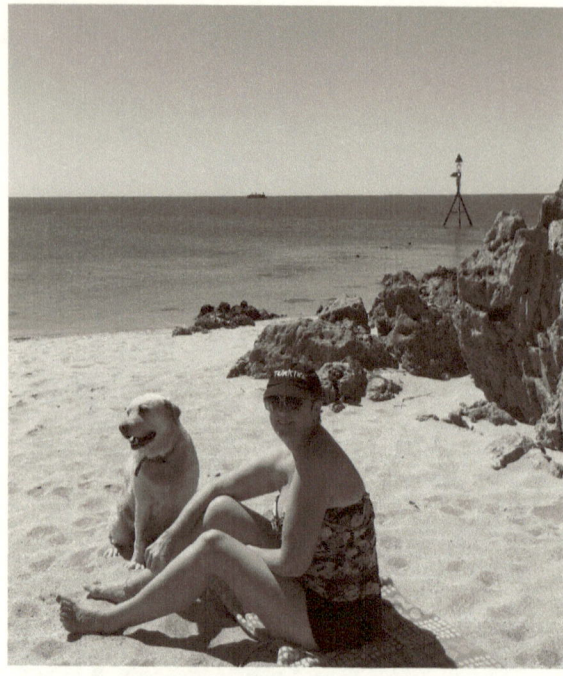

Millie and I enjoying the seaside at Point Samson WA 2016

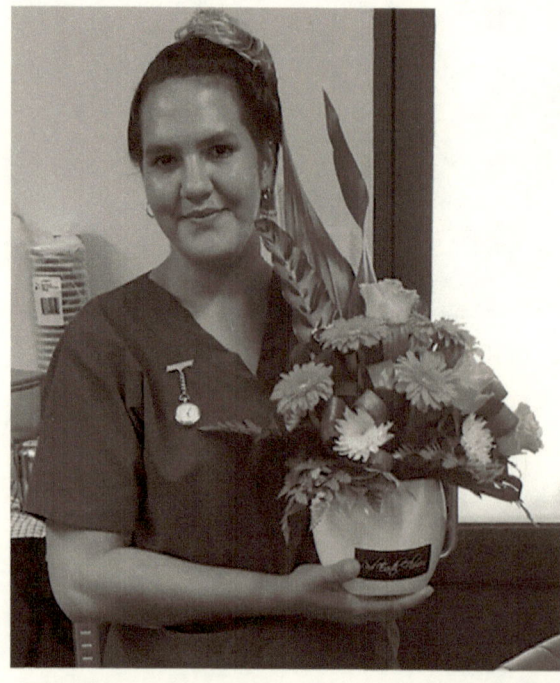

Celebrating Helena's graduation as an Aboriginal Health Worker Mawarnkarra Health Service Roebourne WA 2017

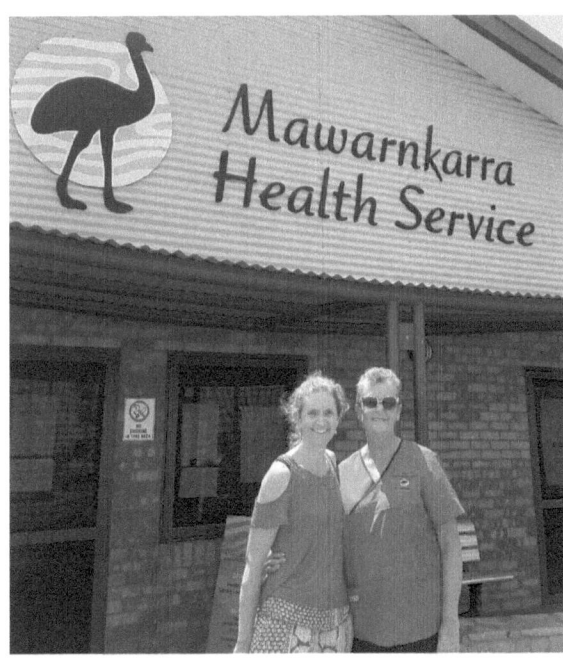

Rebel came to visit, she and I outside Mawarnkarra Health Service Roebourne WA 2017

CHAPTER TEN
Helena

The key to any practitioner, in a new community, is local support. Very early in my employment, I was given the opportunity to interview, alongside others, four people for the role of Indigenous Outreach Worker. Without hesitation, I knew Helena was the one.

Born with cerebral palsy, Helena walked with a limp and had an obvious restriction in her right hand and arm. Despite this, she was immaculately groomed with a stated determination to help her people and to begin her career.

At nineteen-years-old, she knew what she wanted – and I wanted to work with her.

Our patient list was overwhelming; however, Helena and I rocked as a team.

We had so many successes, and the basis of that success was Helena. I learnt so much from her. Helena knew her community. She knew who was doing *sorry business*, what days a home was being used for gambling, where kids were hanging out, who was in trouble with the law, who was vulnerable to abuse and most importantly, who could culturally travel together in the transport vehicle.

First thing each morning, I would give Helena a list of who needed to be encouraged to come to the clinic. Culturally, she would never say no to me, as I was an elder. However, I learnt to recognise her body language.

'You aren't going to see that person, are you?' I would ask.
'No.'

'Why?'

As we built trust, sometimes I got an answer. Other times, I didn't. It was *private business*.

Rheumatic heart disease (RHD) is prevalent among Indigenous children in the Pilbara and Kimberley. This was one of my greatest shocks, as it is now seldom seen in first world communities. The treatment is brutally painful, and resistance to care is high. As a result, children grow into adults with profoundly damaged heart valves.

It is a sorry task to encourage children, teenagers and young adults to present once a month for a thick, syrup like intramuscular injection. For years.

Helena managed to turn our desperately low compliance stats around by contacting the National Heart Foundation and getting posters and photos of healthy hearts and valves, alongside those damaged by RHD. Helena then took visual, graphic information to each of our RHD patients, sat with them and told the story.

I wish I could have taken photos of her sitting in homes, on verandas, by basketball courts and by the river – teaching those young people why they needed to come in every month.

Those kids just needed to feel cared for and spoken to at a level that they understood. Really, that it is often all our patients need.

Diabetes was, and still is, the number one chronic disease among our patients. Left untreated, it sadly leads to kidney failure, sight impairment, heart and vascular disease. Culturally appropriate education was the key to treatment, and our clinic was fortunate to establish an ongoing relationship with Diabetes WA educators, who ran regular community workshops.

We are all born with a certain amount of insulin in our pancreas and in time it runs out. In our non-Indigenous world, that often happens after years of overindulgence in the good things in life, so it is seen as a disease of the obese, affluent and middle aged.

Not so in the First Nations world and certainly not amongst the people I was working with at Mawarnkarra.

We had our own eye-screening machine in the unit and clinic staff gathered one day for an education session. Helena, always keen to learn and participate, volunteered to be the patient.

At the end of the day, screening results were sent through to Perth Eye Institute for reading and reporting.

The news arrived on my desk – poignantly, on Helena's 21st Birthday – that her eyes showed early damage from diabetes.

Tests followed, confirming a diagnosis of type 2 diabetes.

This young woman, like so many others screened, had barely started her life.

Very close to the end of my time at Mawarnkarra, which I had happily extended from one year to four, I had the honour of presenting Helena's story to a WA Diabetes conference in Perth. Helena was far too modest to present her own story, so Ngaarda Media made a film of me having a conversation with her.

I treasure that film, as it represents a story and a relationship that took time and trust to unfold.

It is a story of resilience that should be told.

Helena was born at Meekatharra, WA, on Wajarri Yamatji Country. Population: fewer than 1,000 people. With absolute apologies to the First Nations people who were born in the area, to an outsider, it is in one of the most isolated, dry and desolate areas of WA. Long stretches of tedious countryside pass by in two to four-hours without sign of another settlement.

With little hope of a different life, dysfunction flourishes. Helena was further marked for failure, as she was prevented from playing sport because of her disability. She told me she had turned to drinking and using drugs at a young age.

At fourteen years old, she stood in the main street of Meekatharra and said to herself, 'I don't want this life.'

So, Helena hitchhiked out of her town.

To Karratha, 1,030 kilometres northwest, where she had an older brother with a young family and where there might be hope of change. It would be naïve to think that life suddenly got easy for Helena. However, by nineteen, she was able to drive her own car the 70 kilometres to Roebourne, where she presented herself to Mawarnkarra Health Service as an articulate, well-dressed potential employee.

I can't begin to imagine the strength that took.

During our partnership, Helena was supported in her study by Mawarnkarra. By the time I left, she was a qualified Aboriginal

Health Worker. Nothing comes easy when you live in the vast state of WA. Helena used to drive to Perth for her education blocks, 1,800 kilometres via Meekatharra so she could see family, a couple of times a year. I know that the dysfunction Helena wanted to leave behind is still with her. Helena financially supports family; they are often in her home and the care of a nine-year-old nephew (culturally her son) is now her responsibility.

From my perspective, cultural responsibility can be both a blessing and a disadvantage. There is no denying its relevance in the lives of Australia's First Peoples. The reality is that it can place financial and emotional burdens on hardworking people. The upside is that loneliness and single living is rarely an issue in a culture where family comes first.

If by chance you feel racism in Australia is not a problem, please consider this simple story.

Helena drove from Karratha to Roebourne each day for work. One day, she arrived quite agitated, saying she had to get her windscreen replaced before she could drive home. It had a stone chip from her morning commute. This required a mobile service coming from Karratha to replace the screen. The travel component alone was a considerable cost. I questioned why the urgency, as stone chips seem par for the course – I'd been driving around with them for extended times to be honest.

Helena just looked at me and quietly said, 'It's different for us, Leigh.'

That lovely young woman was terrified of being pulled over by the police. And she would have been because of the colour of her skin.

We both cried when we finally had to say goodbye. I hope an opal from Lightning Ridge provides a symbol of strength and support. I treasure the memory of a tenacious young woman to whom I owe a debt of gratitude for her trust.

CHAPTER ELEVEN
Sandra

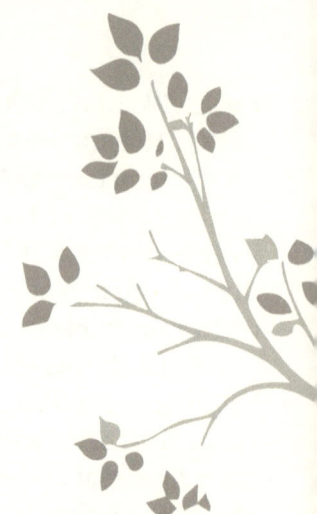

Sandra was a defiant and quite beautiful seventeen-year-old when Helena finally persuaded her to come to see me. Sandra was born with a life-limiting kidney disease to a mum who had suffered appalling, and obvious, domestic violence and masked her lifetime of emotional and physical trauma with prolonged alcohol abuse. There was no lack of love between Sandra and her mother, but Sandra's childhood had not been conducive to the care that she needed to cope with her birth condition. This meant the regular medication that would have lengthened the life of her kidneys had rarely been given.

I quickly realised that Sandra knew very little about her condition and had no understanding of how tenuous her health was as her kidneys rapidly failed. If Sandra was to live, it was vital she continue engaging with our service and with the visiting renal specialist, who serviced the north-west from Perth. In these circumstances, Helena became the vital link. Her search, find and capture skills were certainly put to the test at times.

My three children will attest that I am an advocate of a little tough love and straight talking, and those personality traits were also to the forefront of my initial engagements with Sandra. Trust was slowly developed, and I feel that Sandra responded most to our obvious care for her. Medication compliance was initially achieved by delivering medication to wherever in the community Sandra was on any given day.

Our greatest hurdle to care became getting her to attend the clinic in Karratha to see the visiting specialist, who had Sandra on the books for many years but had not seen Sandra since she was in primary school.

Our service had a long list of renal patients however a very poor rate of attendance at this specialist clinic, despite individual transport always being available through the Mawarnkarra transport service. I gained some insight to the reason when I met the specialist, who asked me why 'a person like you is working in a place like that'. Flying in and out for the day from his place of judgement in Perth, he was perfectly groomed and perfectly representative of non-Indigenous male privilege.

He wasn't the only one who made initial judgements.

In time, I am happy to say we reached an understanding of each other.

'You still here?' Would be his greeting as I accompanied patients to his clinic room. Each time, that greeting was given with increasing respect as Mawarnkarra attendance improved. In fairness to him, I guess he had seen a lot of do-gooders arrive, get burnt and leave early.

During one of our early conversations, the most shocking reality he could confront me with was that none of my Indigenous renal patients, either on dialysis or pending, were on a transplant list. When I asked why, he simply stated they were Indigenous and were not compliant enough. I wondered what sort of dark world I had entered.

I am happy to say this is no longer the case, although, it was in north-west WA in 2016.

Sandra was extremely reluctant to attend the clinic, but I managed to persuade her by offering for Helena and me to drive her to Karratha and stay with her during the appointment. The specialists first question, 'how did you manage to leg rope this one' and the look of absolute fear on Sandra's face indicated we all had a journey ahead.

In the time between having bloods taken and the specialist's appointment, we waited outside, seated on sparse grass under the scant shade of a small Snappy Gum Tree. This was a far more comfortable place than the clinic waiting room for our patient, less so for me.

The kitchen at Mawarnkarra had supplied a light, healthy lunch, which we enjoyed along with the flies and ants. I am sure Helena and Sandra would have preferred KFC or Macca's, both on offer not far away. Come to think of it, so would I, as there would have been tables, chairs and air-conditioning.

Out of the blue, Sandra said that she was 'dreadfully sick for home'. On enquiry, I realised Sandra was homesick for Roebourne, 70 kilometres away, and we had only been gone for three hours. Apart from cultural time out on Country, Sandra had never left her hometown. This made it relatively easy for Helena to find her whenever necessary, but it also left me wondering how Sandra would ever manage the future, which would inevitably involve lengthy stays in the much larger city of Perth, so far to the south, so different in landscape and temperature.

Over my time at Mawarnkarra, Sandra became more engaged with the health services as she realised the severity of her illness and the need for compliance. There was often drama, as the complexity of her life played out alongside her deteriorating renal function.

At fifteen years old, Sandra had been a passenger in a car accident. She had sustained a head injury, which left an obvious scar on her forehead, and there was a pending payment for damages which made Sandra the target for a lot of humbugging from relatives. Sandra would say, 'The Aunties are growling at me.'

Sandra had no fixed abode, no obvious means of income and seemed to survive by couch surfing from Aunty to Aunty. No doubt, some felt she owed them. There was also the concern she may have undiagnosed fetal alcohol syndrome disease (FASD), and her schooling had been erratic to the point of non-existent.

Then, a year on, there was a boyfriend. This was confronting, as the pressure to party with him was intense. Sandra feared losing him if 'she wasn't like all the other girls'. Sandra's blood results, following a drinking session, and her own feelings of extreme lethargy and sickness could not disguise that she was not like the other girls. Sandra's love for this young man was genuine, and her greatest wish was to have a baby to him. She was at a loss as to why she had not conceived.

Those huge brown eyes, her gentle nature and that beautiful young face – with these words coming from her mouth – is enough to make you want to cry for the unfairness of it all.

It was up to a gentle, newly married, female GP to find the words to explain why renal failure and conception were simply not compatible.

In all good teams, there are a range of personalities and perspectives, and one hopes the right person is there for the patient at the right time. It seems that from Helena and my tenuous start to engaging with and advocating for Sandra, the right people were there for her as her health story continued.

There is no long-term, clinic-supported, dialysis in the Karratha/Roebourne area. Patients who want to continue living at home must go to Perth for intensive education on how to attach and operate a haemodialysis machine. First, they need to have surgery to develop viable vascular access. They also require a partner willing to help, learn with them during the training and then support them during dialysis for five to six hours, three times a week, for the rest of the patient's life.

By any one's standards, it is a huge ask.

Years ago, I trained in dialysis care so that I could help a couple of country hospital patients, but to this day, the thought of how vulnerable a patient is when hooked to that machine makes my stomach clench with fear.

I guess when the choice is death, you find your strength.

One of the greatest services offered by Mawarnkarra to their patients is the position of Outreach Support Worker, filled by one dynamic, local born woman named Jodie.

A fierce advocate for the health and wellbeing of our patients, but just as quick to call out any sort of bad behaviour, including, 'smoking, drinking and eating shit food' – no one messes with Jodie, who is based in Perth.

You will find her meeting frightened, disorientated people, who are usually in climate shock, at the city airport with coats at the ready. Jodie navigates her patients to accommodation, organises food and clothing, advocates and often translates for them in the corridors of the health and welfare facilities in which they must spend time.

Jodie is a social worker on steroids.

Sandra's love was obviously not one-sided. In time, her boyfriend recognised her failing health, stayed by her side and ultimately agreed to be with her during her dialysis training. By the time I left the Pilbara, Sandra and he were testing the resolve and patience of Jodie to the limit, but they were in Perth, attending regular dialysis and training. Sandra was also on the transplant list; with the knowledge that compliance was her only ticket to any longevity.

Obviously, her relationship with the renal specialist had improved.

I often wondered how the couple had fared. So, it was with excitement and hope that I read a Mawarnkarra Facebook post in 2022 celebrating their first patient to receive a successful kidney transplant. Facebook Messenger quickly confirmed that it was Sandra. Tears well as I type this.

Successful patient engagement, tenacity, advocacy and care was the foundation for this outcome and is indeed a heartfelt reward for the efforts of many.

PART TWO

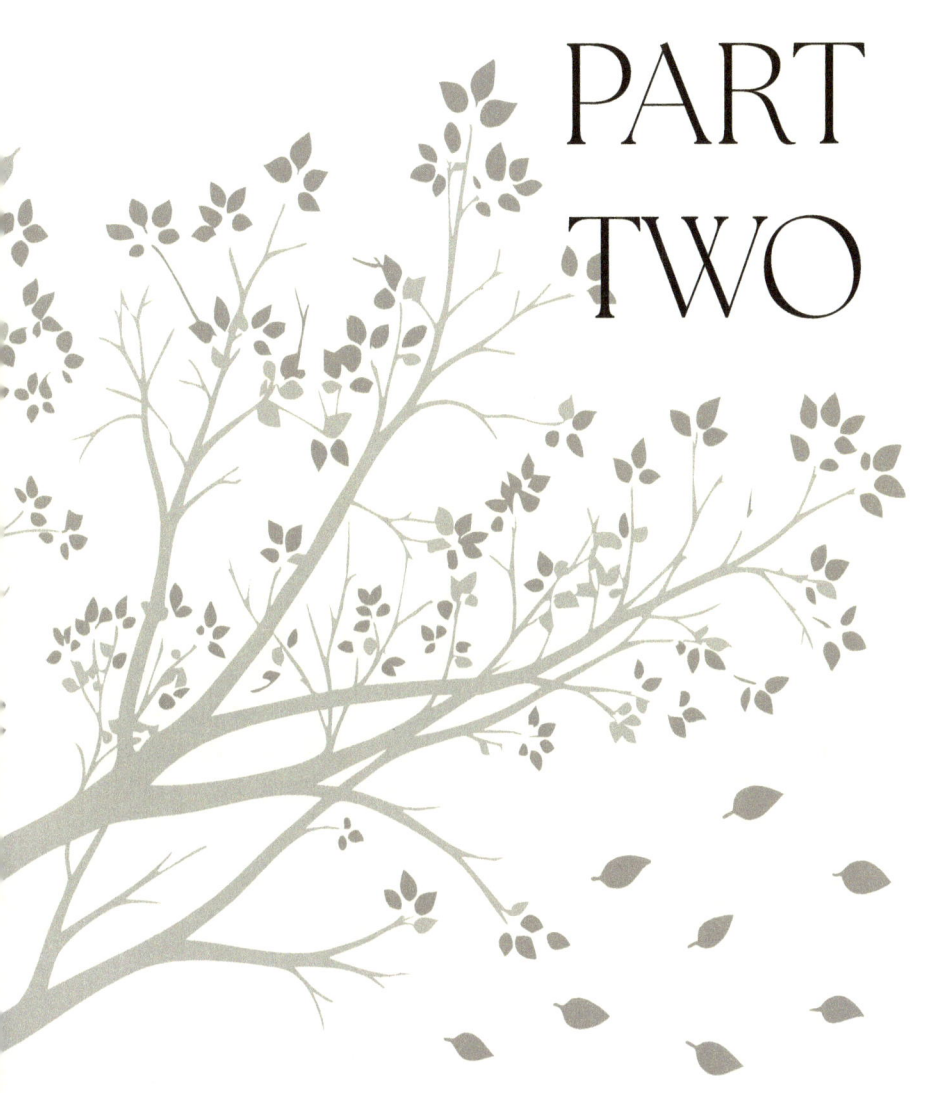

CHAPTER TWELVE
Ricky and Rosemary

Rosemary has now passed. Ricky gives permission for her name to be used; however, he shows cultural respect by not speaking her name.

Their lifetime of love was demonstrated by patience and unconditional service to each other. Rosemary's skin was ebony, her face gentle and her dark eyes soulful. Ricky stands with a confident, handsome presence, always in the dress of the stockman that he is. Rosemary and Ricky met and partnered in their early teens. They had no children of their own but were surrounded by family love and shared responsibility.

About six months before I left Mawarnkarra, a state-of-the-art dialysis unit was opened on-site. Before that, people who had learnt home dialysis but could not carry that out in their homes came to a small room next to my consult room. The room had two crowded dialysis bays, with little room for anyone or anything else, and no window to the outside world.

Rosemary was born on Country. She knew the tree under which she was born and had promised to take me there. During the long hours of dialysis, while Ricky often slept, Rosemary went to that dramatically beautiful place. She was the calmest and most culturally aware woman I have known. Her lifestyle had been quite puritan, yet she still had renal failure. When I met the couple; she had been on dialysis for four years.

Ricky and Rosemary were leading Elders of Ngurrawaana, a dry community just below Millstream National Park on Yindjibarndi Country. In some sort of bizarre swap, Rosemary's people had been given a very harsh piece of Pilbara rock country in exchange for their traditional land, which encompassed the abundant Millstream National Park. Ngurrawaana is about 90 kilometres of rough Pilbara dirt road from Roebourne. Without mains power and with limited water pressure, home was not an appropriate place for Rosemary to dialyse. So, three times a week, they arrived at the clinic for dialysis in whatever vehicle they had pieced together for the trip. Stops for breakdowns and flat tyres were par for the course, treated with humour and a sense of adventure. They seldom had prepared food with them but nothing fazed Ricky, who was a skilled hunter. Both he and Rosemary knew their plants.

During their youthful years, the couple had earnt a meagre income out in the back country hunting dingos for scalp money. 'All those poor dogs,' weighed on Rosemary.

Ricky and Rosemary were an intensely private, independent couple, so it took me some time to realise that they were never given the cooked meals, while in the dialysis room, that the Mawarnkarra kitchen provided daily to all others and through to the broader community. That business took quite a lot of my energy and perseverance to get sorted and I certainly never found out the background to the why. Some sort of interfamily issue, perhaps.

In time, I also learnt that neither Rosemary nor Ricky received any form of social security – no disability payment or carers allowance – and no support for fuel or travel through patient assisted travel scheme (PATS), which is the name for the WA version of schemes, available to patients across rural and remote Australia. These travel assistance programs were established decades prior in recognition of the rural and remote disadvantage in accessing specialist care.

Four years of back payments for fuel was a triumph over bureaucracy for me. The money certainly helped Rosemary and Ricky access some much-needed supplies and cover ongoing fuel and tyres. The social security rabbit hole seemed never-ending.

Eventually, Rosemary accessed payments, but to my knowledge, Ricky never signed off on the paperwork.

'We manage, Leigh.'

Neither Rosemary nor Ricky had a formal education, nor had they ever left their Country before Rosemary's need for dialysis. They were naïve to our systems. English was not their first language, but they were certainly not without intelligence. Four years prior, they had travelled to Perth and learnt the complexity of the dialysis machine. I was never called to their room to give assistance of any kind. They came and went as the days and vehicles suited, but my God, they were compliant.

And here is the kicker – Rosemary was not on a transplant list.

Where was the advocacy when she was diagnosed?

Where was the social worker when the couple were in Perth to learn dialysis?

It was obviously before Mawarnkarra had the funding to employ someone like Jodie.

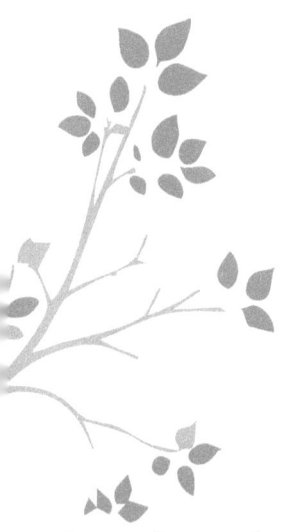

CHAPTER THIRTEEN
An opportunity

One day, early in our developing friendship, Ricky came striding down the corridor with an extra broad grin ... he had been mustering wild bulls and proudly showed me some photos on his phone. He certainly wasn't joking, they were large, feral-bred and their horns were lethal. My adrenaline was pumping just looking at the photos.

For some years of my childhood, and for all my children's, I was involved with horses and cattle. I have a great love of the land and the lifestyle it offers. I had always thought I would love the excitement of helicopter mustering and chasing wild beasts through the bush.

That opportunity, I thought, was long past at this stage of my life.

Ricky expressed despair that the feral condition of his cattle meant that freight to point of sale (1,500ks) took most of any income. He really needed advice from someone who had knowledge and contacts within the broader cattle industry.

My then partner, Andrew, has a fascinating backstory. One that is his to tell. In part, he has been an extremely successful cattle breeder. I had never met a man with such a passion for, or knowledge of, cattle. When we met, Andrew was in a bust cycle in life, charismatic, energetic, with a ready eye for opportunity despite his advancing years. I remember listening to his cattle and WA pioneer land stories and thinking I would have loved to have shared my love of the land with a man so passionate.

As I have learnt over the years, you must be specific about what you wish for.

Always ready for adventure, Andrew had been happy to leave his backpacker accommodation business in the hands of friends to manage and move with me to the Pilbara. His many friends and family were either dismayed that he was too old or excited, and a little envious, of the adventure.

It was only for a one-year contract, after all.

In the first year we were up north, we lived at Point Samson. It felt like a tropical paradise. Having always lived inland, I loved the seaside vibe – our funky, modern home, the high-tide swims, the low-tide walks with my loving shadow, Millie, the kayaking, the fish that Andrew caught, the pub with the stairway to the moon view – and even my bike got some outings.

We loved it all, really – except the midges that swarmed from the nearby mangrove swamps. After Andrew's first day fishing, wearing only a pair of shorts, the poor man suffered the agony of those burning bites and realised why others were dressed from head to toe despite the heat. The itching nearly sent him home to the cool climate of his beloved Pemberton.

It wasn't just that, though.

After two weeks of waking each morning and gazing in wonder at the beautiful, clear blue sky, he looked out the window one morning and stated, 'There isn't a fucking cloud to be seen.'

We had arrived in a vastly different climate and landscape and we both, in different ways, had much to adjust to.

The first few months of my work was quite emotionally overwhelming. I felt the tidal wave of need. Coming home to the seaside, my dog and to a man I loved, who also enjoyed cooking, was a salve for my soul.

Andrew had been prepared to embrace retirement; however, the reality of having a working, professional partner and too much time on his hands was a challenge – he needed more.

Thus began a mutually beneficial partnership between the *old fella* and Ricky.

CHAPTER FOURTEEN
Karratha and Mt Welcome Stations

Andrew was very pleased to help Ricky in any way he could. However, never idle, he had been formulating his own plans while driving down the public roads that traverse Mt Welcome and Karratha Stations.

Recognising that there was limited management of the few cattle evident, and a lot of underutilised country, Andrew thought that maybe management of the stations could do with a consultant.

There is book called *Lonesome for My Country* by Trish Lee, which tells the personal perspective of a young non-Indigenous woman raised on Karratha Station before the phenomena of the mining boom. It is within living memory that the extraordinary rail network, which supports the passage of millions of tonnes of iron ore from Tom Price to the sea at Dampier and Cape Lambert, cut a swathe through both Karratha and Mt Welcome Stations. The development of the rail network, the ports, and the building of the city of Karratha and the town of Wickham forever changed the landscape and lives of those who called it home.

The Ngarluma people hold the land rights to their Country, Rio Tinto holds the primary lease of Karratha Station, and in more recent years, the Ngarluma Aboriginal Corporation has leased back both Karratha and Mt Welcome Stations.

It was into this complex mix that Andrew threw his plan for improvement of both the stations. Little did he know that the current manager had just resigned. In the face of Andrews documented plan of action; he was offered – not a consultant role – but hands-on full management.

A year after arriving in the Pilbara, and at seventy-five years of age, Andrew embraced another dream. Our Pilbara adventure got a whole lot bigger, in fact 900,000 hectares bigger!

It became one of the most challenging and exciting times in both our lives.

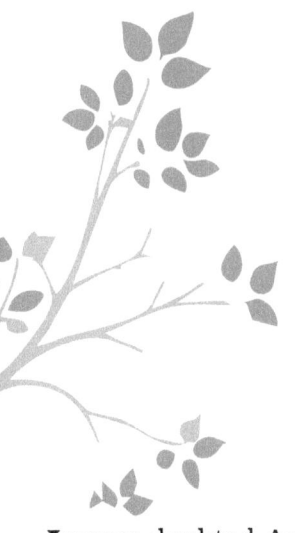

CHAPTER FIFTEEN
Reality

I never doubted Andrew's incredible knowledge, his lifetime of contacts, his tenacity or his life energy. However, I really was concerned about his capacity to get lost in the Karratha shopping centre car park. How was he going to safely navigate his way around those enormous tracks of land?

I shared my concern with Ricky, during a dialysis session with Rosemary. A day or so later, Andrew came home quite angry. Ricky, while showing him around some vast paddock, had tried to send him home in the wrong direction, and Andrew had to argue with him.

'Bastard tried to lose me.'

The next day, Ricky reported to me, 'The *old fella*, he be okay.'

With hindsight, getting lost was probably the least of the dangers Andrew faced.

Little or no maintenance on vehicles, over some years, meant breakdowns were inevitable. The need to carry water with electrolytes was imperative in such a hot climate, and working solo was not wise. A couple of long walks from a broken-down vehicle back to the homestead were necessary to instil some basic OH&S standards in the *old fella*.

Separately, we both knew the challenge ahead would take solid hours of work and enormous effort. We both had prior farming and grazing experience; however, we had been younger then and in more closely settled landscapes.

It was Andrew who had the task.

I could only support him, as he had done me, as I still had my own much-loved but emotionally impacting work to do.

Mawarnkarra had generously met my rental costs as part of my employment package, so we planned to continue living in our clean and orderly home at Point Samson, while Andrew would camp, when necessary, during the week in the grime and chaos of the neglected Karratha Station homestead.

We could have the best of both worlds, enjoying our weekends at either place.

A pipe dream in reality.

CHAPTER SIXTEEN
A treasure chest

Andrew took over management of the stations after an unusually good wet season. There was running water and a good body of new growth feed on the vast spinifex plains. It was fortuitous, as there were very few working bores, fences and mustering yards were in disrepair and internal roads had not been graded for years. Large mobs of cattle roamed and bred at will, they needed time to recover from years of drought and breeding neglect.

Rio Tinto had invested serious money into Karratha Station in the past, so the bones were good. The homestead, a 1970s build on the site of the original stone homestead, was an energy-efficient, modern home surrounded by the old, character-filled station buildings and gardens.

All required a huge cleanout of accumulated rubbish and reorganisation of unknown treasures.

In truth, the whole station was like that.

Andrew needed a truck to transport cattle between the series of cattle yards across the two stations. On one of his exploratory drives, he came across an old Mack on its side about 30 kilometres from base. Ricky recounted that it had been rolled a couple of years prior, on a corner, full of cattle. The driver climbed out relatively unscathed and the cattle escaped. The truck was left.

Pushed and pulled upright, it was well battered, and its brakes were hit and miss, but the old warhorse served its purpose for the years that Andrew drove it.

Andrew wanted to lot-feed the stock he weaned so that they would be of the appropriate temperament and condition for sale. However, extensions to the current yards were cost prohibitive. What to do? He FOUND a complete lot-feed complex. Overgrown with low scrub and well away from public access, it required minimum outlay to bring it back to working efficiency.

Everything which was necessary to run an effective cattle station was there – it just needed to be found and repaired.

Ngarluma management and Andrew felt it was important that he employ Indigenous stockmen, and with Ricky's assistance, he was able to do so.

It was also important to maintain a dry community on the station, which rather challenged Andrew and me, as many boxes of his own wine had accompanied us from its storage in Pemberton.

At the end of our first muster season, a cut-out party was held on the homestead lawn. With memories of shearing cut-out parties, both Andrew and I rather thought the dry might be broken, but no. I have never served so much black tea as I did that night, nor listened to '50s country music at full blast – for hours.

The men provided an ebb and flow of energy for the tasks that were ahead. Working in their own way, Andrew had to adjust to not knowing who was going to be there on any given day. Over the years, those men were a constant source of laughter, frustration, yarns and cultural and environmental knowledge.

I enjoy my memories of puffs of smoke on the plains when the men were out mustering or fencing, burning spinifex clumps to promote new growth in their traditional way.

So many memories.

CHAPTER SEVENTEEN
Millie

On one of my first visits to the station, I took Millie with me. At fifteen, she was an ageing dog but still slim and active, so I thought she would enjoy the space and freedom of the garden. When I opened the car door to let her out, she was strangely hesitant to leave the car and then, would not leave my side.

She wasn't happy.

Two magnificent mango trees stood in the far corner of the homestead yard, surrounded by undergrowth. Andrew disappeared into the scrub, calling excitedly about a discovery, I followed. Millie, who was a step ahead of me, backed away whimpering.

She was quite distressed.

Andrew had found a forlorn and long-neglected graveyard of old pets.

Millie's reaction to Karratha Station unsettled me, and I promised her I wouldn't take her out there to live and most certainly would not bury her there.

Just two weeks later, it was Easter, and Andrew's son and wife had come to stay with us at Point Samson. Both shared a love of fishing and cattle, so we were set to have a great time. Andrew had explored and found a fabulous spot for high-tide fishing on a coastal strip of the station and an afternoon spent there was magical for them, and for me as I went kayaking.

I was silly enough to leave my precious opal earrings on and lost one in the sand, probably when I took off my protective rashie. By the time I realised, there was no sense going back to find something so tiny in such a vast area.

I had more to worry about.

Millie was not herself, and over the course of the weekend, she deteriorated markedly.

While sharing a meal that Easter weekend, with Millie at our feet, Rosemary quietly spoke to me under the radar of the dominating cattle conversation.

'Just love her, Leigh.'

I certainly did that, but by Tuesday, the vet advised euthanasia rather than put her through any further suffering.

It was the first time in our relationship I simply could not fathom Andrew's reaction to my acceptance of that process, despite fifteen years of loving my dog. He couldn't understand how I could 'murder such a beautiful dog'. Andrew would not speak to me for a couple of days before the event.

I slept downstairs with Millie, on her day bed, for her last two nights. A most precious memory. I know it made my outside only dog very happy, but in truth, it was prompted by my absolute hurt and bewilderment at Andrew's lack of care for my feelings.

Perhaps it was an indication of the stress of the task Andrew faced, and his single-minded focus in bringing the stations back to efficiency, which would change our relationship.

Millie was buried, with many shared tears and much labour, in the packed red dirt of our backyard at Point Samson. I placed my remaining opal earing with her as a connection to where she too came from.

Andrew suggested, 'That was a bit generous, love,' as we hugged, cried and then shared a glass of wine to toast our beloved Millie.

That shared burial repaired us, for the time.

CHAPTER EIGHTEEN
Trauma

I do reflect on how we can all become desensitised to trauma when we are young yet grow more emotionally sensitive to it as we age. It has certainly been my experience that my generation grew up with elders who showed little obvious emotion in the face of death or sadness. Boys were actively taught not to cry, and we were instilled with the Anglo stiff upper lip ethos.

A rural life prepares you for the reality of life, death and euthanasia of the rifle kind. I reflect now on the enormous trauma seen by the gentle, loving men in my life, who were at war as young men and then came home to farm, and by necessity, and kindness, to kill animals seemingly without emotion.

To keep those years of accumulated emotion hidden broke them in other ways.

Andrew, with his Italian heritage, was more comfortable with the outward display of emotion. After a hiatus from farming of some fifteen years, he was shocked at how deeply emotional he was when he had to kill his first beast on Karratha Station.

Of the many skills expected of a station manager, killing and butchering a beast, for sorry business gatherings and for stockmen and their families, was a priority expectation. It was a source of pride to Andrew, who had done a butcher's apprenticeship as a young man, to deliver the best on offer. It was certainly his preference to provide a young steer, on request, rather than to find a heifer carcass in the paddock with both hindquarters removed.

That scenario was an inevitable consequence on traditional country so close to a large population base. Keeping a straight face when patients of my clinic described a diet high in beef meat because 'my nephew brings it' was a challenge.

The Future Eaters by Tim Flannery had a profound effect on me as a young farming mother, and the premise of that book is never more evident in the new frontier of the Pilbara.

Pressure from the traditional Indigenous population in Roebourne meant that the people's diet had changed profoundly. No longer were the kangaroos, bush turkeys or goannas in great supply, and the few remaining creatures were actively sought and killed to satisfy an immediate need.

We can be quick to judge others, but before we lose perspective, the enormous scale of mining of the Pilbara landscape seems to me just another form of future eating.

The hunger for the taste and nourishment of kangaroo meat meant that Mawarnkarra kitchen received regular deliveries of western grey kangaroo tails from the far west of NSW – my country.

Once a promise to close gates was extracted, Andrew never denied an Indigenous man the right to access the station country to kill a native animal for his family.

The gates were locked, however, to white fellows who wanted to go shooting just for fun. There were a lot of them – fuelled by big incomes from the mining sector, big toys, big egos – we were not always popular.

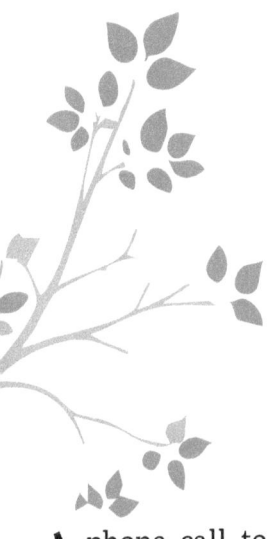

CHAPTER NINETEEN
Muster season

A phone call to the homestead from the local pony club secretary, requesting that her charges be allowed to help with the muster as usual, gave some idea of the level of expertise used in the few years prior.

With mickey bulls sporting lethal horns and temperaments, feral and well-bred free-ranging cattle of all ages, spinifex and rocks over thousands of hectares, a full muster was no place for children on ponies.

Andrew's first season comprised six big musters, involving two helicopters and five bull buggies, with close to a million dollars' worth of cattle sold off the two stations.

So simple to write, not so simple to task.

Months of constant physical work from daylight to dark, along with the demands of management and marketing.

It was a herculean task that Andrew embraced with single-minded focus, great enthusiasm and a lifetime of knowledge and contacts within the WA cattle industry.

With Andrew's safety in mind, and with an inherent love of the land it took only two musters and several potentially dangerous situations for me to release our lovely seaside home and formally set up our shared home on Karratha Station.

Travelling two hours a day for my own work, and supporting whatever was happening on the station, made my life hectic and not without drama. Many of the fluid workforce and families on the station were my patients at the clinic, so the boundaries of work and home were blurred. Dressings, injections and medications were often administered on our back veranda as the sun went down on another big day.

Working with the Indigenous community in the Pilbara was the most respectful experience of my nursing career. Verbal abuse in the workplace had been a given in other communities, but not once while I was in the Pilbara.

Being Elders afforded a level of respect and care that neither Andrew nor I would have received had we not been working with culturally connected people.

My first realisation of the strength and difference of that culture came on Andrew and my very first social occasion in the Pilbara.

A formal ball to celebrate the 30th birthday of Mawarnkarra. Fabulous night. What a party!

The Indigenous country rock band, *Fitzroy Xpress*, had travelled from their homes in the Kimberley (2,242 ks round trip) and absolutely rocked the *Fifty Cent Hall* – as did the crowd! Younger staff reported that the band continued to sing and play all night after relocating to the dry riverbed of the Ngurin (Harding) River.

The lesson, though?

There was to be a crowning of the King and Queen of the Ball.

An assortment of mixed-dress, mainly older, potential winners paraded proudly. My judging, western eye saw no real beauty crowning in the group. I suggested to a local health worker, who was young, delightfully willow of build and quite beautiful that she should be up on stage.

'Shame,' was her horrified reply.

My lesson was well learnt when the crowning winners were judged.

Two elderly people who had spent years working in a voluntary capacity in their community and who were much loved and respected. *Shame on me.*

When I moved out to the station, one of the men asked me, 'You like being yelled at missus?'

'No, this missus doesn't.'

'Does the old fella yell at you?' I asked

'All the time, missus!'

I was to learn another side to my beloved partner.

In the early 90s, I attended the very first NSW Rural Women's Conference where Christina Hindhough was a keynote speaker. Christina was the sister of an admired ex-prime minister's wife, Tammy Fraser, and had just published a book called *For better, For Worse and For Lunch*. This book had become a bible of sorts for a generation of young farming women who were pushing the boundaries of their male-dominated environment.

Christina strode on stage and, with great presence asked, 'Why is it wherever I stand in the sheep yards, it is the wrong place to be?'

Eight hundred women roared with laughter, many of us cried, 'We were not alone!'

To this day, I wonder how farming wives are immune from the principals of workplace bullying and abuse. I hope it is different for a younger generation.

The three years Andrew and I shared on Karratha and Mt Welcome Stations are a kaleidoscope of quite extraordinary memories – most wonderful and a few challenging –which will always fill my heart with gratitude.

A top favourite was being rewarded for hospitality by the pilots of those tiny muster helicopters.

'Want a ride?'

I loved it.

Never mustering, as that was too dangerous, but I enjoyed several flights to fuel bases and one memorable adventure ride with a young man whose off-season job was as a driver of the *Shotover Jet* in Queenstown NZ. Quiet lad but definitely an adrenaline junkie.

Another favourite, when time allowed, was assisting with the muster in my very own bull buggy. Queen of the plains was I. Youthful dreams do come true.

Andrew and I shared a lot of adventures and occasions which we would have thought we were long past. The pinnacle of those was the Fitzroy Crossing Bull Sale.

Prior to leaving on the 2,400-kilometre return drive, Andrew commented that we would probably stand out because we didn't have a pair of long boots, belt buckle, tight jeans or large cowboy hat between us. I suggested we would stand out for another good reason – we were pretty old!

I have always loved the adrenaline and dust-filled atmosphere of a good cattle sale but hadn't been to one in many years.

OMG, this sale was top-end, big bull, cowboy porn.

We did stand out for reasons other than age and dress, but not before we were ignored by a couple of known agents who were busy currying favour with potential buyers. Never been prouder of my man because Andrew, with the backing of the Ngarluma Board, had a very deep pocket that day and, with his astute eye for quality and workability, made a series of top bull purchases.

Andrew, the Ngarluma Corporation name and those top-of-sale-bulls made the news and no commission to agents needed to be paid. We were feted that night by several very happy stock breeders in the best, and only, restaurant in town, and therefore in full view of the agents.

Rather an *up yours* moment on a few levels.

Scenically, the stations were a glorious landscape to live, work and explore.

Sunday afternoon drives for a bore run, cattle check and a swim, in a newly discovered waterhole, became a highlight of the week. A magnificent wonderland for the adventurous which we were able to share with a constant stream of friends, family and people passing through.

Many of those visitors contributed invaluable extra hands during the muster season and in return for the cleaning up, catering, mechanical and cattle-handling skills shared, I trust they were rewarded by a unique experience and taste of station life.

Andrew and I loved the company.

Drinks on the veranda, or on our favourite rock hill, with its panoramic views of a setting sun, was a rich reward for a long day's work.

A couple of our visitors were of questionable value, however...

I well remember a rather lengthy camp on our homestead lawn of a knockabout mate from over east. Turned up with his new girlfriend, and her very large dog, while on a caravan journey around Australia.

He had always worn a cowboy hat, told tales of his youth on Kimberley stations and had maybe done a few too many brain cells in his time. You may know the type – heart of gold, on a pension, after a free camp and enjoys a few beers.

Day two, 3 pm set up on the homestead lawn, stubby in hand, he is asked if he would mind helping load the last of the feral cattle, from the eastern yards, which were to be carted some 40 kilometres to the main station yards. The stockmen, not reliable at the best of times, had gone to town as muster season was over.

'Yep, no worries, the girlfriend will come too!'

First, though I – who was staying home to cook the evening roast – was asked to tow the truck as it needed a jump start.

Why?

It was the old Mack that had been found on her side out in a far paddock. Battered, with limited battery function and no lights, she worked well unless she stalled, or it got dark.

Off they all went.

Peace surrounded me for a few blissful hours, but then it got dark, and darker – no moonlight that night to light those vast plains. The roast was well finished.

What was happening?

My mobile rang – my heart pounded.

'Are you OK?'

'Yes, love, but I can't see a fucking thing, only one bar of service, no torch, no water – it's in the work ute – can you come and get me?'

'Of course, but where's our mate?'

'Don't know, he just kept driving, and he knew I had no lights.'

Out I go to the shed, get a reliable vehicle (mine!), water and a torch.

Twenty kilometres down the dirt track, I came across the girlfriend and old mate by a gateway, sipping on a beer, leaning on the work ute.

'Where is Andrew?' I ask.

'Don't know,' came the reply. 'We've been waiting for him to catch up to us.'

'He hasn't got any lights on the truck mate.'

'Oh!' Blank face.

Girlfriend digs him in the ribs.

'I told ya that.'

Unimpressed, I left them to it and drove on to find the stranded truck, with two decks of feral cattle bellowing, and a very thirsty, happy to see me partner.

With my car headlights showing the way home, the truck right behind my precious car, is another story – I did say the brakes in the truck were not reliable.

My car was regularly in use to rescue or transport, its suspension and duco took a battering, but it was reliable, and I often fuelled up from the station tanks as recompense.

One day, I was taking a couple of older stockmen to town, and we drove past the construction site of the new Karratha Hospital. I commented how good it was going to be to have such a wonderful facility.

'Five hundred sheep drowned in that paddock in the 50s,' came a voice from the back seat. Karratha is built on a floodplain.

I do wonder if Australia's First Peoples historical knowledge and advice were ever sought – probably not.

CHAPTER TWENTY
Spirit world

Rosemary was about fifty-eight when she died, in her seventh year of dialysis, which is about as long as the body can cope with the assault of dialysis. She knew her time was coming as she was becoming weaker. I was back east for my son and daughter-in-law's engagement party, and my mother's failing health, when Andrew rang to tell me the sad news.

I love that Rosemary had spent the night before her passing at Karratha Station, on a patch of lawn outside the stockman's rooms, lying on her swag under the stars, with her man.

Ricky has a brother, Frank, who loved the tiniest little dog named Shorty. The three were constant companions, once Rosemary died, as Frank too had lost his wife at a young age.

Just on dusk one evening, I pulled up at the southern cattle yards about 30 ks from the homestead. The air was thick with dust and the bellowing of newly mustered cattle. The two helicopters were just airborne, headed to the homestead, weary men were packing their gear into the bull catchers. As I got out of my vehicle, Ricky and Frank, with Shorty in his arms, came over, excited to tell me about a miracle that had occurred.

Shorty had been tied up in the cabin of their vehicle but had managed to reach the window and had launched himself out in a bid to get to Frank – effectively hanging himself. At that moment, Frank happened to glance over to his vehicle from the yards from which he bolted to his precious pet.

Holding him in his arms, he howled. 'He is dead, he is dead.'

Ricky, only a couple of paces behind, snatched the tiny creature off his brother yelling, 'Stop saying that! He will hear you and believe you.'

As Frank recovered from the shock of his brother yelling at him while he was grieving, Ricky actioned full CPR on Shorty. And there he was, in all his bug-eyed wonder looking at me from Frank's loving arms.

Spiritual connection to Country lives in the soul of Australia's First Peoples.

The longer I have spent with the people on Country, and the more open to the wonder of the energetic universe I have become, the more the country and its creatures have spoken to me. Never more so than in the Kimberley and the Pilbara where culture remains so active. In our western way we listen to our gut, have a sixth sense or just bowl on through those feelings in our haste to go forward.

As my time to leave Karratha Station drew close, Ricky kept Rosemary's promise to take me to the place where she was born.

An exquisite and pristine waterhole, surrounded by paperbark trees and low-lying red dirt cliffs. It is an understatement to say it was quite a trek to get to. Our vehicles took a battering as we traversed rocky ridges, wide plains and deep waterways. Closed to the adventuring public and inaccessible most of the year. What a privilege to share such a day with Andrew, Ricky, Frank, two close friends Kath and Stuart, and of course Shorty.

While the men yarned, no doubt about cattle, Kath came with me as I felt the need for some quiet time and a private soak in the pool. While my friend sat as sentry, I waded through reeds and into that beautiful water. As I paddled, soaking up the ambience, a magnificent black cockatoo glided down in front of me, turned its head, looked straight into my eyes, then turned and flew off.

I was deeply moved.

When the opportunity arose, I told Ricky.

'That be her.' he said.

It is important for my physical and mental wellbeing to walk in nature, so every morning that I awoke on Karratha Station, I walked a short way and then climbed to the top of some huge, red rock outcrops which the homestead is nestled by. The view over the vast plains to the south was my reward and I was often joined by soaring eagles.

On my very last morning, I climbed.

My heart was heavy as I stood, looking over the view of the plains, homestead and the outbuildings.

My contemplation was interrupted by an eagle, of vast wingspan, flying from my left, past me, at face level – so close!

As it passed, it turned its head and met my eye before flying off.

I had been bid farewell.

My time there was over.

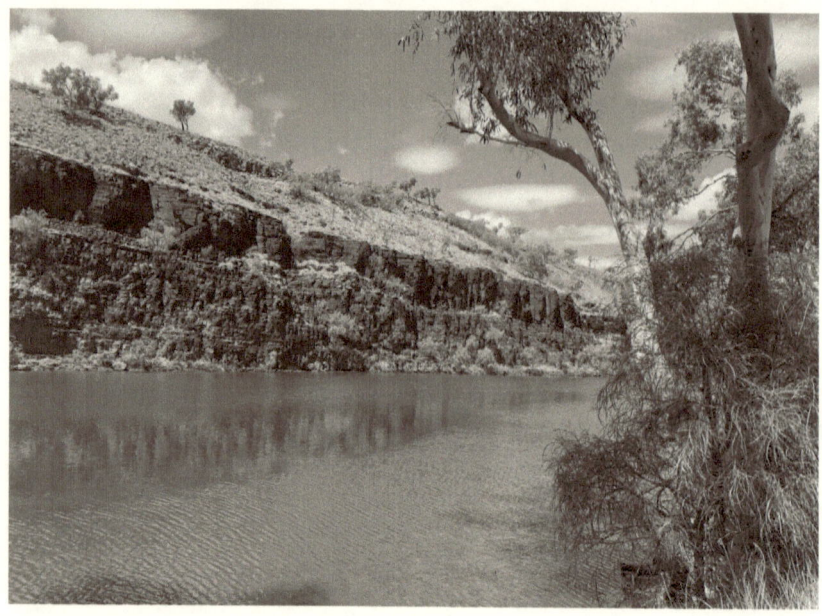

A favourite water hole for kayaking Pilbara WA 2016

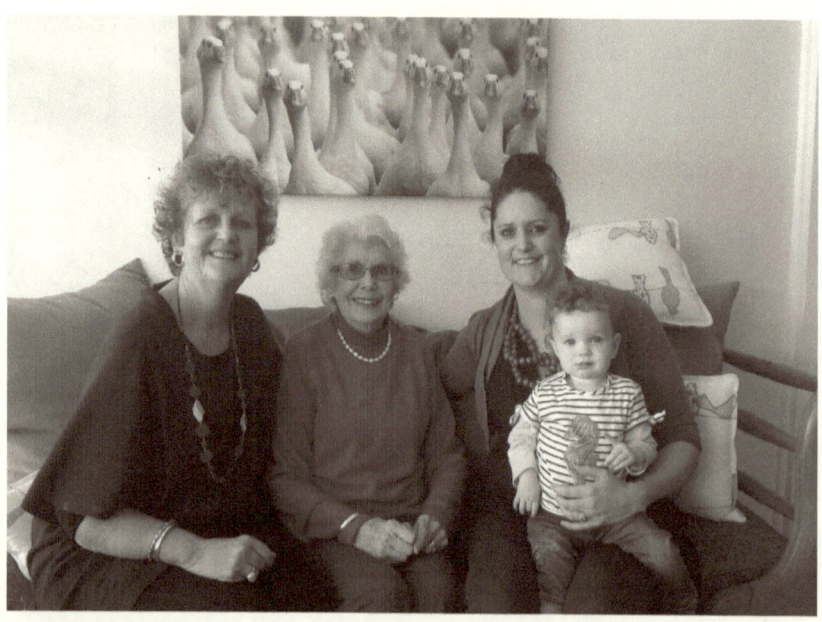

Four generations of maternal love, my mother Gwen, daughter Deanne, granddaughter Montana and I Coonabarabran NSW 2016

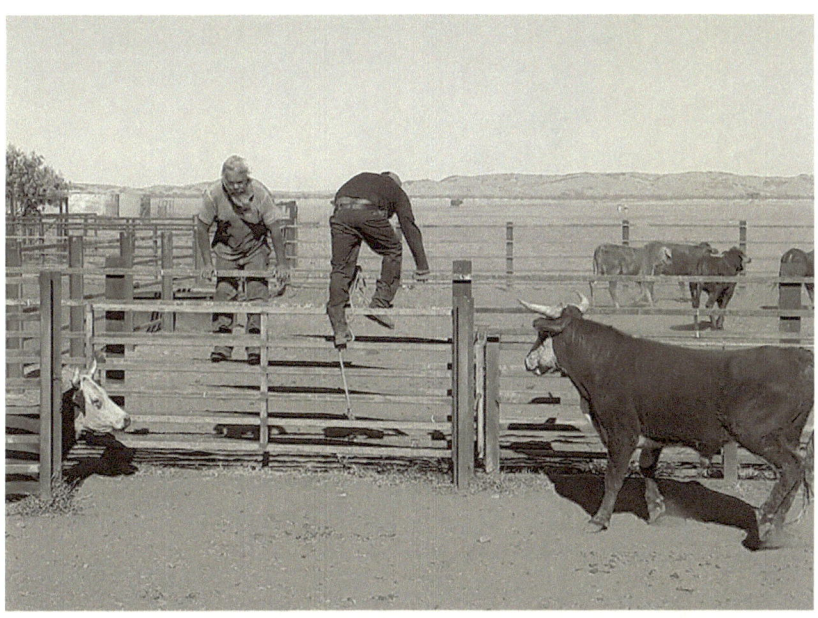

The yards were not a safe place to be Karratha Station WA 2018

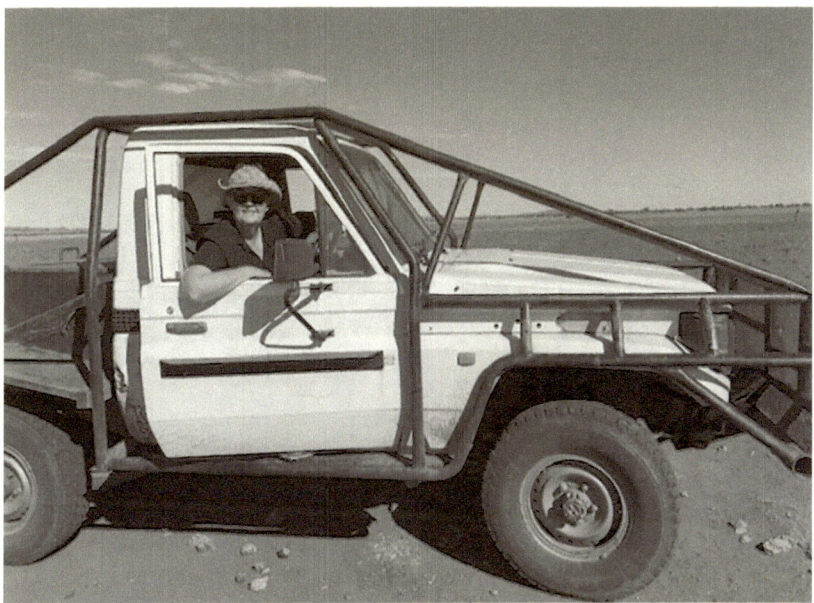

Adrenaline boosting fun mustering with one of the bull buggies
Karratha Station WA 2018

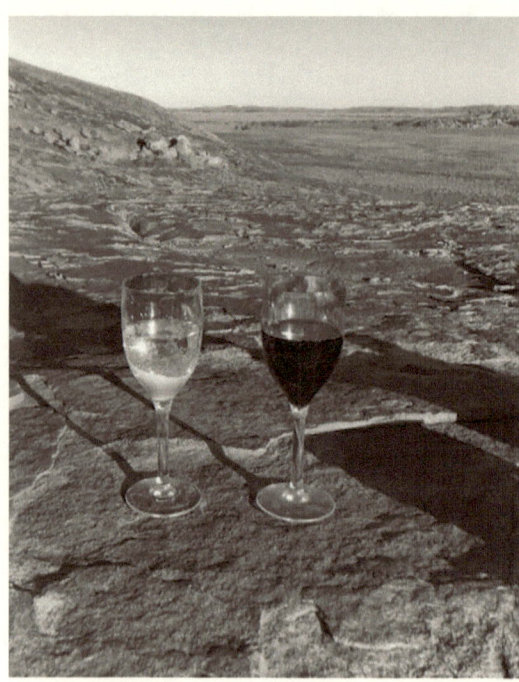

Pilbara red rock
sunset drinks
Karratha Station
WA 2018

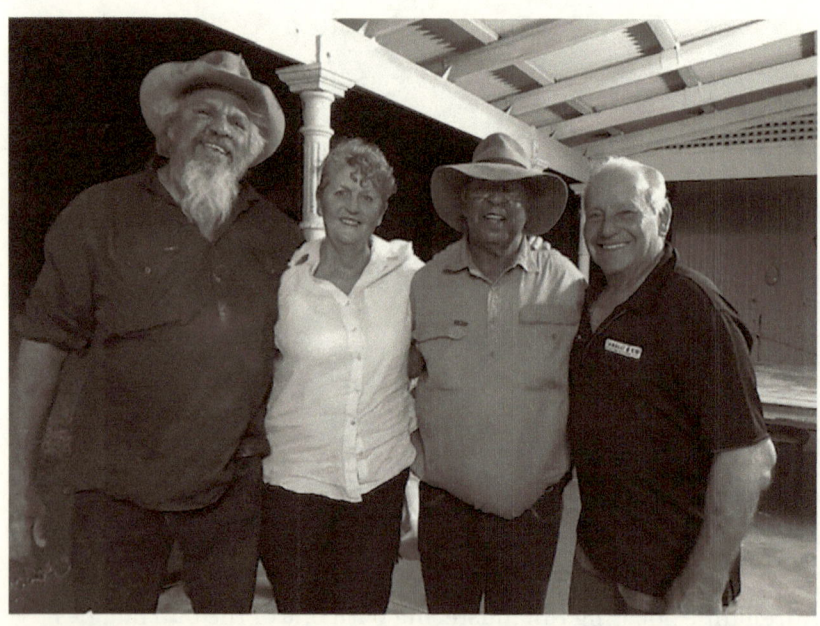

Ricky, Frank, Andrew and I Karratha Station 2018

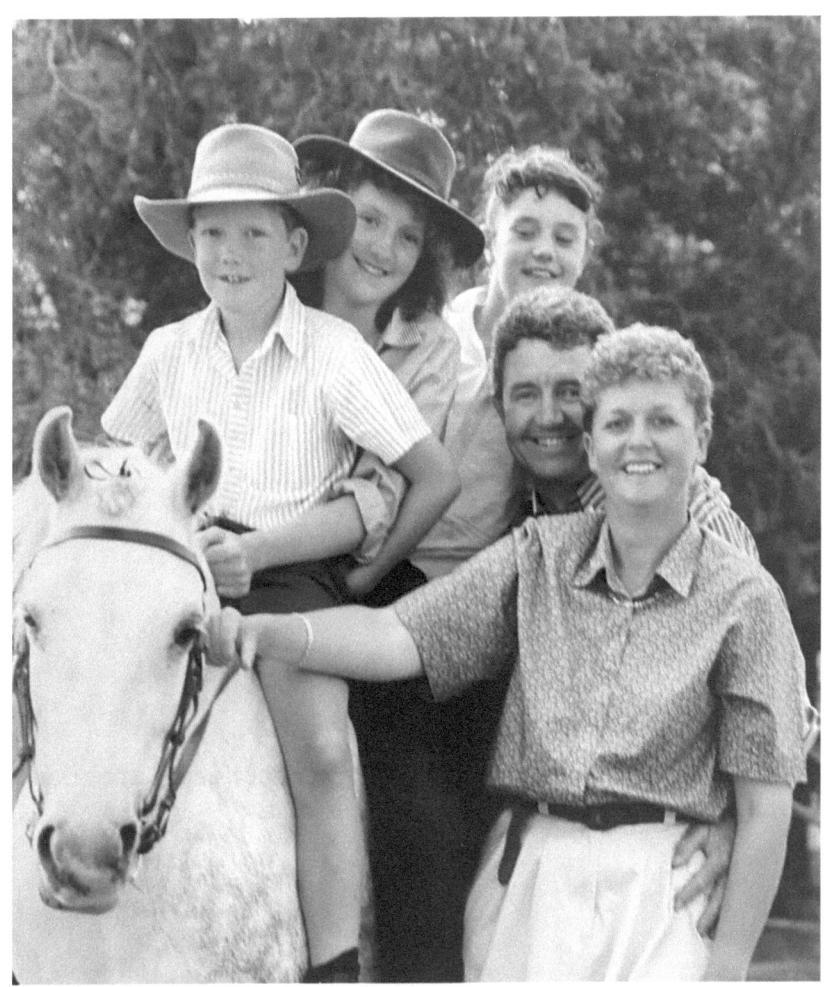

Calypso the pony, Cameron, Rebel, Deanne, Rick and I on our family property Purlewaugh NSW 1988

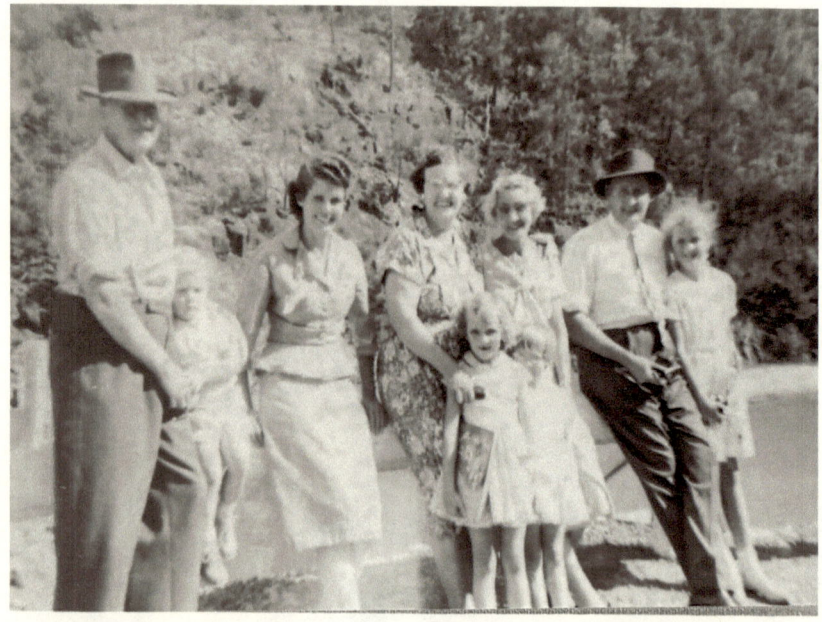

My family before my father and grandfather's accident Timor Dam Coonabarabran NSW 1963

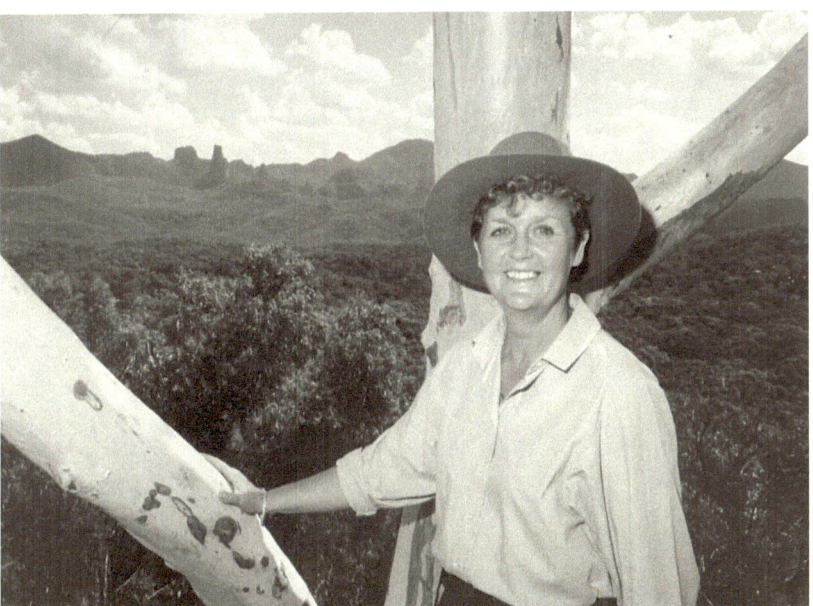

My favourite place:
White Gum Lookout Warrumbungle Ranges

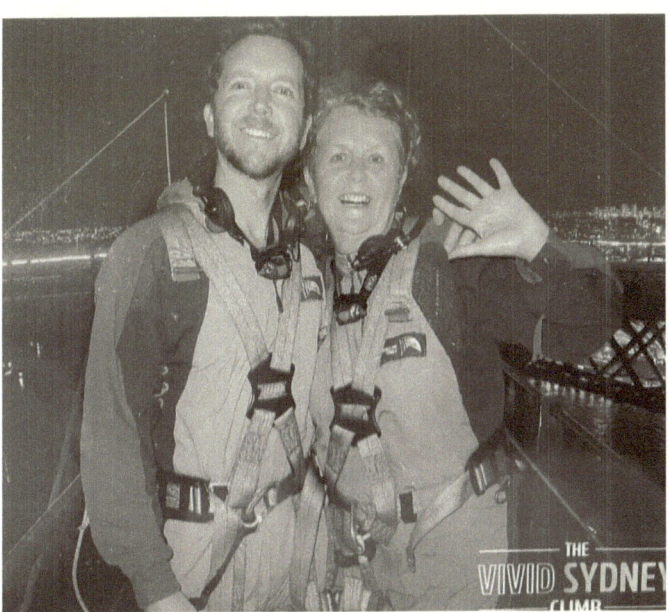

Cameron and I celebrated his 40th and my 70th by climbing the Sydney Harbour Bridge

PART THREE

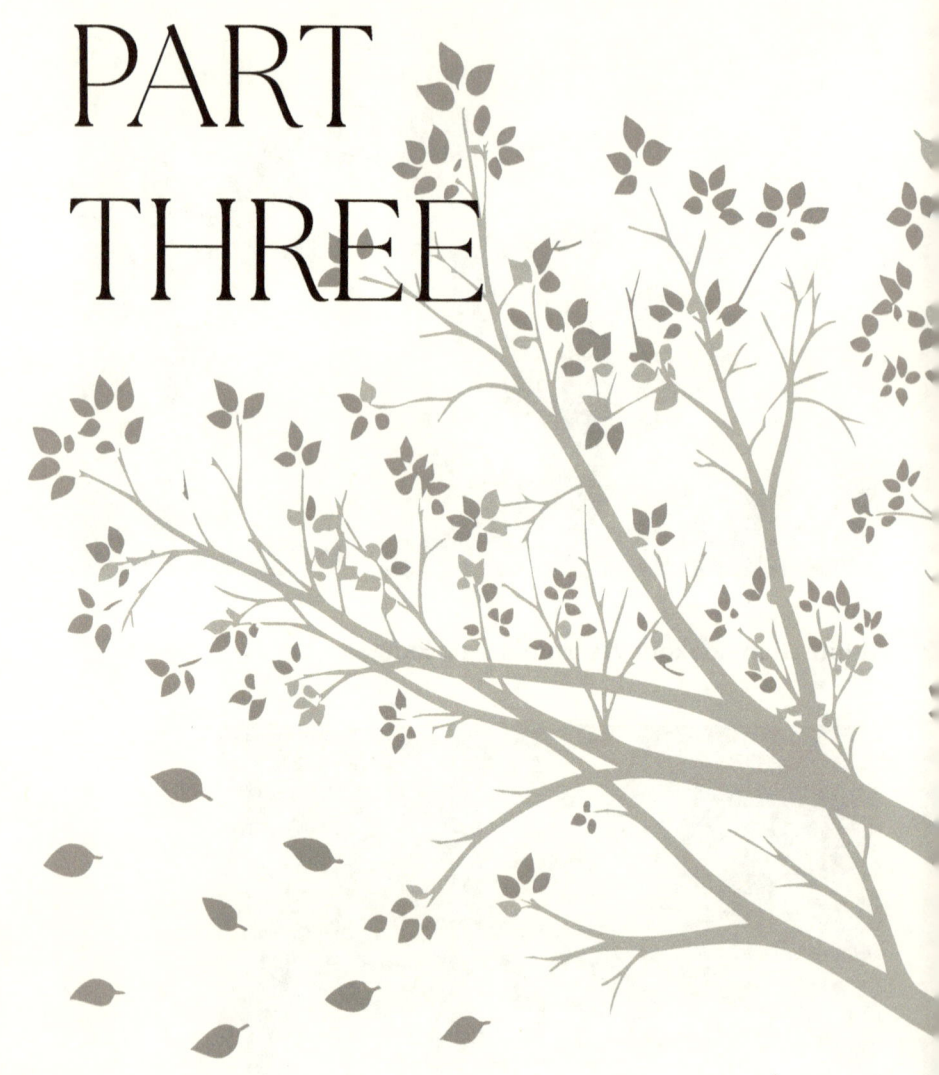

CHAPTER TWENTY-ONE
Why a nurse?

In my sixteenth year, in 1968, I relied on the generosity of a farming family east of Moree, in the Pallamallawa district, for the provision of a home and the ability to complete Year 10. I was a straight A student and a confident participant in school life. I would have loved to continue with my education however my family circumstances did not allow that. Prior to any form of social security support, I sat an examination for a Commonwealth Scholarship however was not successful. Another path was needed.

My caring host, Mrs Keam, had been a registered nurse prior to marriage. You will note that in that era it had been deemed 'inappropriate' to continue nursing after marriage, or pregnancy, so there were many young nurses relegated to the exclusive role of housewife and mother. In fact, nursing was seen as excellent training for that role with the extra titillation that one might have advanced sexual knowledge!

It was Mrs Keam who suggested that I should apply to Royal North Shore Hospital, Sydney, to commence my training. In support of interview success Mrs Keam took me to the 'best' clothes shop in Moree and chose a lovely pale blue, linen A-line dress for me to wear. Such a generous and thoughtful gesture for which I hope I showed gratitude. My clothes until then had been handmade either by my Mum, or increasingly, by myself so I recall I felt very glamorous.

At the end of the school year, I bid a tearful farewell to a crowd of school friends, and my Keam family, on the platform of Moree train station. I waved until they were out of sight, however, my tears took longer to dry. There was one very fit young man who hugged me at Moree station, hopped on his pushbike and cycled the 20 miles to Gurley Station, to which the train had slowly travelled to again stop for passengers. We managed another hug. We have not seen each other since and I doubt he ever knew how much that hug meant to me.

The combination of my smart dress and academic and school leadership record saw me interviewed and accepted into Royal North Shore Hospital however not until I turned eighteen in 1970. That year of waiting, living in Sydney between generous god parents and my increasingly unhappy family, was essentially a very lonely one as I knew very few young people. I filled my time and my savings account by working as a chemist assistant during the day and as a waitress in the evening at the first Italian restaurant on the North Shore of Sydney. The very popular Puttini's in Gordon.

Toward the end of that year, I met Paul. A kind and decent young man who became a confidante, and my first lover, until he was called up to serve in the Australian Army. Like so many of his generation his active service in Vietnam forever altered him and like many young women I did not have the words or the knowledge to love and support him on his return. I recall I was in second year nursing and living in a share unit when Paul's final term of active service ended. Under cover of darkness, to protect from protesters, his plane flew into Sydney Airport and disgorged its uniformed cargo of young men into the arms of waiting families. I was on night shift and Paul met me as I came off the ward. I covered my uniform with an overcoat, but Paul's uniform was obvious as we walked through the city streets to my unit. As we came up the stairs a horrible old neighbour sneered 'been out on the town all night, eh?' I had never witnessed the anger that Paul exploded with as I dragged him away from the man and through my front door. Paul was sobbing, 'You have been saving lives, and I have been defending our country'. He was furious!

Our relationship ended in time but not before attending a wedding I have never forgotten. In the early 70's virginity at marriage was deemed desirable thus very innocent, white gowned young women were walked down the aisle by proud fathers. The bride of the day had no idea that her husband, fresh off the plane from Vietnam, had an active venereal disease he was too scared to tell her about! Hard to imagine now, though I am sure such ignorant deception happens.

In March 1970, I commenced my nursing training one day prior to my eighteenth birthday. Surrounded by 35 other young women, I doubt any of us had any idea what we were to experience and I wonder... if we did know would we have chosen a different path?

I recall much excitement as we were kitted out in our starched linen uniforms, assisting each other to navigate the correct way to pin and pleat our aprons and caps from which my curly hair never failed to escape! The excitement of being shown our tiny single rooms in Vindin House Nurses Home – mine with a view to a church spire in the distance. I was to see many a bleary-eyed sun rise over that spire!

Our first six weeks were spent in Preliminary Training School (PTS) with the first practical lesson being the correct method of mitring a sheet corner when making a bed. Rulers were in action as top sheets must be turned down four inches. I was to later learn that a newly made bed could be stripped in anger by a ward Sister, ruler in hand, and a junior nurse humiliated in front of her patients if that rule was broken.

Early in PTS we were asked if we wanted to know what shifts were to be worked. I was naively astonished to realise that PTS would be the last block of time that I would work 'normal' hours: night shifts, early morning and late evenings were to become our new normal. We quickly learnt the rigid hierarchy of hospital training where anyone who was even six weeks ahead in training must be stood for when they entered a room. My mother said the discipline of nursing would be good for me however I don't think that even she would have approved of the fear that some of that discipline caused. I believe that it often sabotaged curiosity and individual thought as we were confined by so many rules and restrictions.

I quickly realised how very fortunate I had been to be accepted into Royal North Shore Hospital as I was the only girl in my group who had not graduated Year 12 and therefore, I was amongst the youngest. I was also one of the few who was not privately educated and who was from the country. Also, my attractive mother was again single, with a young family and working successfully in the, then, male-dominated world of real estate. Curiosity about my family's difference, in that conservative world of the time, was a fascination however it did set me apart. I do know now that my tough times have made me empathetic, and I often think it must be hard to have empathy when nothing much has gone wrong in life.

Our year of commencement, 1970, was the start of nurses completing their hospital training in three years so for some years we were in the presence of women with four stripes on their caps. We revered the capacity of those young women as we set to the tasks of a junior nurse – pan room duty, day room duty and ward tidy nurse being the role of nurses without any stripes. It is no surprise that our patients loved us, and often confided in us, as we were attending to their most basic human needs and I feel they often felt sorry for us as we worked hard in open wards that housed up to 50 patients at a time.

With hindsight we grew up very quickly once we were on the wards. One's first experience of the vulnerability of a body with multiple injuries, the intimate workings of the human form of all ages, witnessing death, the sight and smell of necrotic wounds and body fluids, all impacted and there was no such thing as support or debriefing for a nurse traumatized by such experiences. Those who had a romantic image of caring for others were often amongst those who chose other career paths early in their training.

My first death experience was of a Registered Nurse who died a slow death of lung cancer. Just after 10pm it was my sorry task to accompany her, with a trolley orderly, to the morgue, which was a rather scary, long, torchlight walk from the ward. Back in the nurses' home, just after 11pm, I shared my first half packet of Craven A cigarettes with some of my friends. The irony is not lost on me!

My first injection was given to a lady, a private patient, who complimented me on the administering of same. I was so proud that I blurted 'it's my first time but I have given them to cows before' she was not impressed. It still makes me laugh!

On that same private ward there was a man in a single room who felt he had licence to touch any junior nurse in any way he felt compelled. It took one brave nurse to go to the senior nurse on the ward who then questioned a group of us. We had all experienced the same humiliating behaviour so, six nurses, led by our senior nurse went to the office of the charge sister. Despite our leaders articulate recounting of the problem the charge sister dismissed us all stating 'what rot; he never does that to me!'. Chastened we exited the office and outside the tension was broken by the senior nurse saying, 'why would he want too? she is old!' That fellow's bad behaviour stopped when he had an unfortunate incident; someone put effervescent Dexal in his urinal prior to use.

It's an old trick.

Very restricted budgets and the threat of termination of training if one was caught at a party with drugs, or if one was unfortunate enough to fall pregnant, was a deterrent to excessive drinking, drugs and sex. There was still a lot of fun to be had though! One of the most counter protective measures in place was the hospital policy of locking the nurse's home at midnight and reopening it at 6am. There were no room welfare checks so if you were not home by midnight you simply had to find somewhere else to sleep unless you had the foresight to apply for a 1am or 2am pass. You were only allowed such a pass if you were on a day off, or a late afternoon shift, the following day. At the given times of 1 or 2am there would be a sorry line of young women in various states of dress, inebriation or exhaustion, sitting in the Central Sterilizing Unit awaiting the stern gaze of the night sister before being escorted across the hospital grounds to the home. Many a young man risked licence and safety, driving madly to get girls back in time to meet curfews and many young women were made vulnerable by just staying out and sleeping on a party floor or in the back of a car. It is no small wonder that most of us were anxious to organise our share rentals by the time the first year of compulsory 'living in' was over. It was a shame really as there was a wonderful, shared camaraderie in the nurse's home with the added benefit of cleaners, linen supplies and three meals a day. However, freedom is a temptress!

Three years of training flew by in a heady mix of youthful energy with few boxes left unticked by the time of graduation! Without the two years of higher school education the science of nursing eluded me however the practice of nursing, responsibility and care held me through my exams – no subject was ever failed however it was a close call at times. Graduation Day – the wearing of a veil, the receival of the prized hospital badge – was a day of celebration, pride and relief!

CHAPTER TWENTY-TWO
Sliding doors

In 1975, fuelled by confidence in the assurance that a training from Sydney's Royal North Shore Hospital would open doors to constant employment in my chosen career, I approached the matron at the small Coonabarabran District Hospital in northwest NSW.

After graduation in 1973 I had spent time specialling private patients in the eastern suburbs of Sydney, where I witnessed a sharp contrast in wealth and privilege. I then worked in the recovery and surgical wards of the Tamworth Base Hospital. At the time of approaching the matron in Coonabarabran, I was living in Sydney and had commenced my Midwifery Certificate at Hornsby District Hospital.

My focus was on a career in rural nursing, where midwifery skills were necessary, and I was in love with my young farmer, Rick. I imagined sharing a life on his family property in the fertile Purlewaugh district east of Coonabarabran.

Imagine my surprise and distress when I was informed by the matron that she would never employ me.

She gave her reasons as: 'you are marrying a farmer, so you will not need the money and you will not be reliable, as you will be living on a dirt road.'

That sliding door moment and the ignorance of youth.

Why didn't I look at her and realise that she was old, that change would occur, and I had my working life ahead of me? Under pressure from traditional farming family attitudes, I accepted that my future husband and the farm came first and six weeks later I resigned from my midwifery training. I was blessed that before leaving I had a couple of wise senior midwives who supported me in fast forwarding some of my delivery skills so that I might be better prepared in the event of an emergency delivery. There have been many occasions when I have blessed their foresight.

Of course we needed the money.

With the benefit of hindsight, that 'old biddy' did me a favour.

I did a crash course in touch typing after being offered work at a local legal office. One year spent there was a great introduction to accounting, legal practice, office management and speed typing, all essential life skills for an efficient farming wife.

A year later, a new matron at Coonabarabran District Hospital, Miss Knapp, changed my life path back to nursing.

Another newly graduated registered nurse and I were called to help the older nursing staff set up and learn to use the first cardiac monitor in the hospital. I clearly remember the call to the legal office from Nappy, as she was fondly known, 'What the bloody hell are you doing working there?'

The times were changing.

The 'old biddy' was right though, about my potential for unreliability on dirt roads!

I recall many days of having to stay in town due to impassable roads, having my vehicle and me towed behind the tractor to get me out onto the main road, of many a slip-and-slide drive in the most amazing little Datsun 180B – bright orange and as game as I was to go where it may have been wiser to hesitate.

I only recall being late for one night shift.

Unexpected rain was falling heavily as I left home very early, thinking I could get out for my 11pm shift. Dressed in my white uniform, stockings and sturdy shoes, I was driving the farm ute, which Rick had told me might get through the rising waterways more safely. The change of vehicle proved a disaster. About two kilometres from home, I went into a slow, free mudslide and semi-rolled into a deep gutter. Naturally, the emergency pack I had in my trusty Datsun was not in the farm ute – so no torch, no two-way, and long before the era of mobile phones.

In fact, we were still on a party line with its Morse code signage.

Pitch black night, pouring rain, sloppy, slipping mud. I climbed out of the ute, clawed my way up the bank and walked home. They say you know a road like the back of your hand. I proved the expression right that night. I slipped often however the only time I misstepped was into a wooden ramp – that horrible falling sensation into a dark pit – fortunately shallow, but to add to the sorry picture barked and bleeding shins. There is no part of this story that is exaggerated, so you can imagine the horror on Rick's face when I stumbled through the door! Phone call made to the hospital, shower had, scrapes patched. Clean uniform, back in the Datsun with the tractor in front, dragging me to the main road.

Yes, I was two hours late that night, but please don't think me unreliable.

CHAPTER TWENTY-THREE
Family time

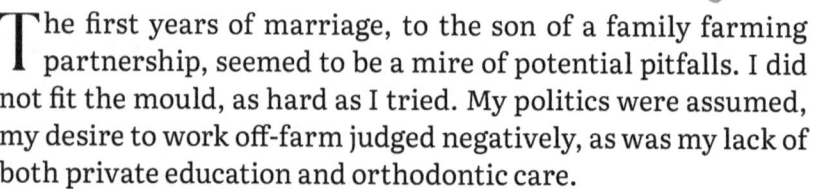

The first years of marriage, to the son of a family farming partnership, seemed to be a mire of potential pitfalls. I did not fit the mould, as hard as I tried. My politics were assumed, my desire to work off-farm judged negatively, as was my lack of both private education and orthodontic care.

Worse still it seemed, in a conservative community, my attractive and resilient mother had been widowed, remarried (a bigamist, as it turned out) and then had recently married again to our wonderful stepfather.

At work, the judgement continued.

I recall a team of us about to lift a patient onto a theatre trolley. As the registered nurse in charge, I commenced the count – one, two...

'STOP!' The commanding voice of the GP anaesthetist.

We all stopped, looked, as he directed his gaze on me.

'Are you pregnant, Sister?'

'No, Doctor.' My red-faced reply.

'Well don't leave it too long, no farmer wants an infertile female on his property.'

The transfer was completed in stunned silence.

Fortunately for all, infertility was not an issue. However, before starting a family, Rick and I wanted to spend time together away from the responsibility of farming. Rick had come home to work with his parents following one year of university and eight years at boarding school. We were still only in our 20's. With his parents' absolute disapproval but resigned consent we enjoyed three wonderful months travelling in England and Scotland in a hire car, Europe in an 'under 30's' bus with serious mechanical issues and a final two weeks in Greece. My savings had paid the way, the budget was as tight as it could be however it was the most wonderful time of adventure, misadventure and freedom.

We arrived home pregnant with our first child and committed to our life choices.

Three precious children: Rebel, Deanne and Cameron, were born, and I embraced my evolving role in the farming partnership. Well before childcare was available, I did try to nurse night shifts when the children were very small. Balancing sleep deprivation, the children, travel time and the demands of a farming and grazing business proved impossible and so; my nursing career was put on hold for fourteen years. I will be forever grateful for the flexibility of our life, then, which allowed us to nurture our children in what, I believe, to be the best of growing environments.

Dozens of family photo albums are a reminder of the abundance of memories that our family are blessed to hold. Three children in four years ensured sibling playmates who were surrounded by a variety of animals, space in the natural world and a mother who was able to take them most places while contributing to the farm workforce. There was little need for toys and make believe as the real thing was just outside.

Perhaps their father and I pushed a bit too hard at times; I recall Cameron as an eight-month-old in a cardboard box on the back of his dad's motorbike with his two sisters on the front, me on my horse, while we mustered sheep. Going down and out of a gully the box fell off... sickening fear, never forgotten... Cameron crawling out of the box with a grin of approval for the bumpy ride!

A playpen, under the shade of a Kurrajong tree, full of toys, books and my little ones as I drove a tractor, ploughing around them in ever diminishing circles.

Truck driving was my main task when the children were young – they could off course come with me freighting livestock or produce. I had to get my heavy vehicle licence first and that required learning to double clutch for gear changes. Dressed in my best 'town' clothes I failed the first extensive examination on a minor technicality. Two weeks later I dressed in my working clothes and with a more 'butch' attitude a second examiner simply required I drive around the block to succeed!

Christmas 1982 was very dry, and we were hand feeding sheep. A grain bin was on the truck with a shute at the back where Rick used to precariously balance and control the flow of grain into long narrow feed troughs. It was important to keep a steady and accurate flow into the troughs as the sheep could smother each other in their weakened state of hunger. We had been working all morning, it was hot, the girls were sick of the truck and Cameron, a baby, was hungry.

One more paddock to feed out. Popped the girls over the fence with strict instructions to stay close by and to watch mummy and daddy feed the sheep. I started the truck with Cameron nestled in the crook of my right arm happily breast feeding, all going well until one of the girls got scared and they both started screaming. Their dad, yelling at me to ignore them as the sheep were stampeding into the troughs, me trying to drive the truck to instruction while feeding! I do recall yelling back at Rick 'Happy Christmas to you too'. An evening invitation to our closest neighbours was a welcome end to that weary day. We sat on their veranda, surrounded by those who understood, watching with hope as some distant storm clouds gathered. I love the word 'petrichor'!

Our family grew with horses, farm animals, bikes, 'paddock basher' vehicles and space – there were prangs and some broken bones however all possible care was taken to have quiet animals and a sense of responsibility and respect for both the animals and the machinery. Some of the very best memories our family share as adults involve working in the shearing shed, stockyards, mustering and then every year Pony Club and competing in our local show circuit.

The school bus run each morning, and afternoon, scheduled and shaped our lives. Two hours travel a day for the children with drivers they spoke of with reverence – and the mischief that was made! Rick and I were very happy to provide an old blue ute for Rebel to drive the five-kilometre dirt lane way, to the bus stop, when she was twelve. Quite old enough to take responsibility we thought – and thankfully she proved to be!

The most 'out there' act by our children was to decorate their ute with colourful emblems of peace, goodwill and rainbows. Parked on the side of the main road, for the duration of the school day, it was deemed by a conservative neighbour 'unsightly and it lowers the tone of the area'. From then on, the vehicle was parked more discreetly in the yard of a dear man, Murray, who lived about 500 metres down the lane. We thought it an exceptional vehicle as it seldom required attention. It wasn't for some years that Cameron casually informed us that Murray frequently did running repairs on the ute!

For a time, I thought I would never go back to nursing as other opportunities arose which better suited our family situation. I gained a position on the first female only Rotary Group Study Exchange to the USA in 1988. It was a big deal as it was prior to Rotary accepting female membership. In a significant move, for that time, Rotary also accepted my status as a Farmer and Grazier. I recall being questioned about the welfare of the children in my absence. I was proud to assure that the children had a father most competent of their care. There were raised eyebrows.

It was an exciting chapter in my life as that opportunity opened possibilities and connections in the marketing of wool products into the USA.

Before the internet and prior to Australia embracing the concept of product liability insurance; my dreams required financial backing and more time, when the wool market crash happened.

I went back to drenching sheep – but only for a while.

My next thought was to establish a tourism business as I had experienced, while in the USA, the interest in my family's lifestyle and we lived close to an established tourism market. With the need to supplement our wool loses Rick was strongly supportive, and with our growing children's assistance, we thoroughly enjoyed some years of touring and offering hospitality with Coona' Country Tours. I am very aware that would now not be a politically acceptable name. In defence, it is what Coonabarabran and district residents call their town.

The tours afforded our family happy memories, and I know that we provided special memories for all our guests. One of our saddest scenarios was the most memorable.

Our children, and other district children, had learnt to ride on a gentle natured, hairy little pony named Twinkle. Cameron was her 'last' child, so she enjoyed a long retirement in our care. On the day that was to be her last we all said our tearful goodbyes as it was time for the children to start their bus run, and I needed to collect my tour guests; Rick was left to see Twinkle through her last hour.

Toward the end of the tour, which went through our property, I noted smoke from a funeral pyre, explained the situation to my guests and apologised in advance for the inevitable family emotion. Stopping at the homestead, as the children pulled up in their ute, required only a nod from me and there was cascade of tears and hugs with the guests ignored! Those city folk later told me it was one of the most poignant and loving scenes they had ever witnessed: they had never thought of how attached to an animal a family could be when there were so many others in the paddocks. They were most grateful to be shown 'real life'.

One of the most fun things we did during our tour era was to host bus groups into our shearing shed which had, with poor timing, been renovated and extended just prior to the wool crash. Bernie, ex-shearers' cook and raconteur, catered hearty baked dinners with Nan's apple pies, doused with lashings of custard, for dessert. Bernie's wife was named Nan, so he had no hesitation in saying that the pies were Nan's 'home-made' however we needed to have the cardboard evidence well burnt, on the outdoor bonfire, before the bus came up the laneway! Music was provided by a talented father and son duo, Wilf and Tony, with a shearing demonstration by one of our local men, Craig, who was an excellent shearer, appropriately attired, full of good humour and respect. A change though when Craig arrived for evening shearing demonstrations! Humour, talent and respect remained however tighter pants, cut off shirt sleeves and the certain strut of a very fit young man ... the ladies loved him, and he played the game well!

During the worst of droughts and after the wool crash, while Rick and I balanced the property, tours and the needs of our teenage daughters and Cameron, who had developed a rare and often life-threatening illness, I also worked three days a week with funding from the Department of Rural Industries. The grandparent collective became of vital support.

At a time before rural counsellors were established, and at the beginning of rural aid initiatives, our small team generated a great deal of money into our community and were of support to many. I am very proud of the work that we accomplished - it was exhausting and heart-wrenching and by far the craziest, busiest time of my life.

All that was done off-farm cost money in fuel and vehicle wear. Those many kilometres travelled are a reality for farming families and often go unrealised by those who live more urban lives. We were blessed with beautiful countryside to travel through, and travel time provided talking time or time to de-stress from one list of chores and refocus on the next list!

There was the odd flat tyre, ran out of fuel once, but only one accident on a long straight stretch of the Purlewaugh Road. It was dark, travelling home, Cameron in the front and six dozen eggs on the back seat. It had been a busy day at work, I had forgotten to drop the eggs into my parents and Cameron, and I were to drive to Sydney for his medical care early the following morning.

I was driving our Toyota Landcruiser which had a sturdy 'roo bar on the front. A black steer was suddenly under our headlight beam, close, I swerved into the oncoming lane however the beast ran across the front of the vehicle, I hit it front on, full force at 100ks, we were so fortunate to have been in that solid vehicle. I was able to back off the beast, which was still alive, and park off on the correct side of the road. On opening the back door, a cascade of broken eggs poured onto the roadside. A neighbour came up behind and stopped to help as I had my hazard lights flashing and head lights on.

While I called for help on my two-way, she and I discussed how to put the poor animal out of its misery. Within minutes we saw headlights coming at speed toward us and toward the black beast lying right across their side of the road! We were about to witness a real accident!! I frantically flashed my lights on and off, on and off, the driver didn't slow, just dropped his high beam thus diminishing his sight! We were all driving the right cars that night ... a low Subaru outback hit the underside of the beast as if a ski jump, flew into the air, pieces of undercarriage shearing off and hitting the road with sparks flying, and down the straight miraculously landing on all four wheels, the car slowly turned and drove back to us. It was surreal! Craig the shearer, all six foot four of him, climbed out of the Subaru and said, 'What the fuck was that?!' 'A steer, you hit a steer' 'it's dead now' 'we need to get it off the road!'.

'But there must have been chooks here – there are eggs!!' We were all in shock! I called Craig Geoff on the night, which is his brother's name, for which I have been teased however I rather think I have the upper hand with his reference to chooks!!

Through those years our children were awesome, competent, resilient young people. Cameron's health settled in time however while in the acute stage it challenged our family's strength and resources. I have never been so grateful for my nursing training which empowered me to ask the questions and to care for, and advocate for, Cameron during his frequent hospitalisations. Masking my own distress became an artform!

There are two stand out memories that I wish to share from those years – both in the first acute stage of his illness; Cameron required emergency blood transfusions – his first received in Dubbo Base Hospital to stabilise him to allow for air transfer. He was only twelve and acutely unwell. I thought our children had been sheltered from the years of horror of the AIDS epidemic. The ability to screen blood for the virus had been developed the year before. As that life giving blood came down the IV line to enter my precious boy, he turned his head to me and said, 'Why are you trying to kill me?' a king hit from which I did some fast nursing, mum talk! Our family had a wise woman in our lives who visited Cameron and I while he was at the Camperdown Children's Hospital in Sydney. A regal presence, Elizabeth came to Cameron's bedside, picked up his hand, turned his palm up, pondered for just a moment and said, 'My you have a long lifeline Cameron', put his hand down and started to chat to us both. After she had left Cameron said, 'I am going to live Mum, Aunt Elizabeth said so'. So simple, so powerful!

We would not have survived those years without the ongoing support of a wonderful rural community, caring medical professionals, school, family and friends. The expression it takes a village to raise a child epitomises our family's experience. It was a grand village!

It was possibly inevitable that at the end of my child-rearing years I made the decision to return to the nursing profession after a six-week refresh at the College of Nursing in Sydney. I remember the pleasure of being back in the company of nurses as we share a special bond and humour.

Inevitably perhaps too, our marriage collapsed with Rick's decision to sell our family's home and beautiful property. Something broke in me the day Rick announced his decision, he looked so happy and relieved, it was his right to make the decision however the lack of consultation devastated me. All that we had worked for! All that I loved! I knew instinctively neither of us deserved to live with the anger and distress that I felt. Our marriage was over. I was emotionally shattered.

I acknowledge now that Rick had lived my dream and his father's – not his own, which is a lesson, in its way, to all those who work in the succession planning business and to generational farming families.

CHAPTER TWENTY-FOUR
Grief

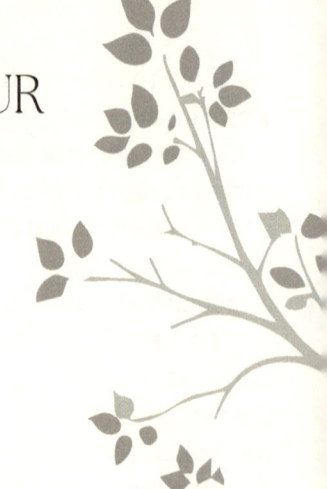

My heart country is the Coonabarabran district, in Gamilaraay Country, New South Wales.

My early childhood was spent on acreage, in a lovely home my father, a builder by trade, had built in the Hills District of Sydney. When I was nine, and we were a family of four very young children, Dad fulfilled a life dream by purchasing a 5,000-acre bush block on the edge of the Pilliga State Forest, north of Coonabarabran.

It was not a wise financial decision.

At the time, Dad was a partner in a real estate business in Liverpool (now a city in the Sydney basin), when all the land surrounding was being developed for housing. I recall going with Dad to the British migrant hostels nearby as he negotiated land sales. The 1950s in Australia was an era bursting with possibility and population growth. 'Populate or Perish', they said.

Brought to an isolated, tiny cottage at the end of a sandy bush track, with only generated power and tank water, I have no doubt it was a very tough time for our mother. Those 5,000 acres however, afforded me the very best of childhood memories – before tragedy changed our family's life.

My Dad and Grandad, those wonderful First and Second World War veterans, 40- and 70- years- old, were killed in a car-truck collision some miles from the iconic outback town of Bourke, in far west NSW.

I was eleven at the time.

My sisters, seven and five, and our baby brother three. My mother a widow at thirty-six, my grandmother a widow at fifty-eight.

At the time of death duties and long before there was any government support for a grieving widow with four children, my mother showed remarkable courage, independence and resilience. In that stoic, Anglo cultural way we got on with it and the children were protected from the grief of funerals or any conversation about either of the men.

It seemed to me that they were forgotten.

I reached a mental health crisis when I too was thirty-six and was fortunate to have wise counsel – it was then that I truly grieved the deaths of my father and grandfather.

One of the tasks of grieving that I was given was to blow up a balloon, write all my feelings onto the balloon and release it to the heavens. One of my favourite places on earth are the soaring peaks of the Warrumbungle National Park. Only an hour's drive from home I thought it the perfect place to let go. On the anniversary of my dad's death, my children and husband were aware of my task so, I was solemnly hugged and off I drove with water, picnic snack, balloon and a Texta in my backpack.

I planned to climb the Grand High Tops with its panoramic view of the great western plains. The climb is not for the feint hearted. I got to the top about midday and dutifully blew up my bright orange balloon, then proceeded to write my feelings through free falling tears.

Prepared to let go; there was not a breath of wind. The imagery of floating away was changing, maybe I could throw it over the edge? No, it plopped down in front of me. I threw it harder, no, it sat on a ledge. I retrieved it, threw again harder, nearly went with it, it plopped to a lower more precarious ledge, now the tears were replaced with anger, then laughter as I retrieved it and realised that I could kill myself trying to get rid of my grief feelings! Belatedly, I then realised I couldn't, in all conscience, litter a nature site, so I popped the balloon, scrapped a hole, buried it and placed a rock over it.

The lesson for me: the intensity of those feelings might decrease each time they are outed however they don't ever go away!

I did however hike back down the trail with a lighter step.

Life hack: another task, which I found profound, was to write a letter to my dad with my non-dominant hand. It opened a pathway to my inner child, and that little girl poured her feelings on to pages with childish scrawl. I burnt the letter as part of the process but have never forgotten the release I achieved.

Under supervision, it is a wonderful tool for anyone dealing with childhood trauma.

Just two years ago, my son Cameron and his wife Jess, their children and our family suffered the death of a full-term baby named River. The way that incomprehensible grief was expressed and experienced was in direct contrast, for me, to the way of previous professional and personal grief experiences. All those years of hiding from death, of taking a baby away, of sheltering children, of not talking about feelings, all has changed so much and even though it was confronting for me, at the time, it is so much for the better. Even language. At the time of mourning River's death, I sat on the lounge with his four-year-old brother, Cooper, and told him how sorry I was for him that he had lost his baby brother. With an astonished expression he looked at me and said, 'Oh Grandma, I didn't lose him, he died!'

Out of the mouths of babes.

Our Anglo culture has so much to learn about grieving. It is one of the starkest contrasts when working for First Nations people. Again, I bring it back to the personal experience.

My beloved stepfather, my children's only known maternal grandfather, died in the early hours of the morning, in Coonabarabran. Four hours' drive away; I received the news and immediately made plans to be with my mum and extended family. First, I went to my office and did a day of work so that I could leave my responsibilities, before sharing those few sad days with my family. The day after the funeral I drove to Bourke, for a work commitment, the place of my father and grandfathers' death all those years before. I do recall feeling that was so wrong... fucked to be honest. In contrast, one of my colleagues, for whom I have great admiration, had his mother die on Country in the Northern Territory and he did not come back to work for three months. Sorry business, as it should be.

On return to Karratha Station following my mother's death, I recall the way Ricky and Frank held me close, a group hug, they keened, I felt their energy and grief as a vibration. I couldn't bring myself to let go as much as they – I wish I could have.

The laying out of a patient was a precise skill base when we trained as young nurses. I remember supporting a senior nurse with the task for an elder Italian man while his family waited impatiently on the other side of the curtains. I was slower than my colleague in getting out of the way, once the curtains were pulled back, and was enveloped in what seemed a communal embrace of grieving hysteria as the family rushed to our perfectly wrapped patient. I was pushed back onto the bed and body and literally had to slide down and out through those poor people's legs.

My demeanour and precisely placed nursing cap took some adjusting.

There is more sensitivity now however cultural misunderstanding is very real.

I learnt a lovely lesson in rural nursing early in my marriage, at the deathbed of an elderly neighbour. I was on an evening shift when the gentleman passed, surrounded by family, with his dear wife holding his hand. My professional demeanour was shot to pieces as tears poured down my cheeks. I went to bed that night feeling ashamed of myself for not holding it together. The next day I was on shift when the son came for his father's belongings. I quietly apologised for my show of emotion. He was gracious enough to share that his mother, while having a cuppa with her family, had reflected how gentle her husband's death had been, how special and loving it was, and that 'even Sister Black had cried'.

It is not easy nursing people you know in a community in which you have your roots. It isn't always easy for them either. Issues of privacy are paramount. Trust and respect are hard won, and one misplaced word or deed can undo years of goodwill.

Thus, like so many professionals in small communities, I kept many secrets and distressing incidents from my husband and obviously from my children. I know it was not healthy for my marriage, as my husband remained naïve to many facets of my being and life experiences.

CHAPTER TWENTY-FIVE
Self care

The nursing experience of witnessing and listening to trauma events, while also living one's own life, carries an emotional burden and for many clinicians causes mental health problems. My own mental health has been sustained, in part, by a decision, very early in life, to not let any one person's actions stop you leading a good life – a don't let the bastard get you moment.

I also read *Pollyanna* by Eleanor H. Porter as a child. Published in 1913, it tells the story of a young girl who always found something to be glad about, even when life was hard. A prelude to our modern concept of gratitude. That practice has served me well, as has my love of the natural world and my access to it.

My journey from accident and emergency care to chronic disease management, in my mid-50s, was prompted by a developing essential tremor of my dominant hand. Exacerbated by stress, I was very mindful that as a registered nurse in an isolated workplace, I could well fail to negotiate a procedure, requiring fine motor skills, if a patient or family were yelling at me to do something.

But what else to do?

By chance, I had not long before done the high-altitude trek to Macha Picchu in Peru. A life-affirming, but perhaps foolhardy decision, as I was then 20 kilos above my healthy weight and had done no mountain climbing for years ... and never any high enough to tip you into altitude sickness. Toward the end of each hiking day, when fitter hikers had reached the campsite, one of the young porters would come back to me and take my 7kg backpack. I felt SO light with that weight off and could almost skip into camp.

The lesson was not lost on me as I returned home determined to lose the equivalent of three backpacks and get fitter. I took long service leave, went to the Gold Coast, south of Brisbane, Queensland and trained in Certificate III and IV in Fitness. My classmates were young, buffed and beautiful, and when asked by the lead trainer why I was there I did wonder myself. My fitness learning became my personal journey and thus I became a personal trainer. At the end of the eight weeks of training, I was offered a position as a fitness coach, for the elderly, in a range of elite Gold Coast aged care facilities. However, my heart was still in remote care, to those less privileged.

As often happens in life, a decision is made to change, and the universe provides.

On my return to Lightning Ridge, I was having coffee with a past colleague who commented on how well I looked, I told her about my new fitness qualifications. She said, 'I have a job for you.'

Thus, my career segued to chronic disease management in the western region of NSW.

Aside from the professional advantage, the daily practice of finding joy in movement has meant that I have enjoyed many more adventures since, it has supported my good health and, most importantly, it has supported my mental health.

There is nothing like a good walk in nature to sort your thoughts.

Nature always teaches:

In an emotional recovery phase, post-divorce, I recall lying on a towel-draped sun lounge, in my swim costume, by a pool in the grounds of a motel. The time and peace of the moment felt like luxury, I was writing my annual Christmas letter on a pad, supported by my bent knees. Deep in thought I felt a pressure under my left thigh, not looking, I put my hand down and tugged lightly on my towel. I felt a prolonged slither under my left thigh and up over my crotch.

I looked down, straight into the eyes of a large brown snake, tongue flicking, head slowly moving side to side. I froze. I continued to stare, as did the snake, it seemed for minutes but probably only seconds, and then it curled back over my crotch and slithered under my right thigh, down off the sun lounge. As its head reached the grass its tail, on the other side, left the grass and all that time, I remained frozen. As it slithered away into the garden, I started to write about two words and then the adrenaline hit. I shook for some time, showered diligently, burst into tears and then, once sympathy was delivered, had to field phallic jokes from the friend I phoned.

Laughter is, after all, a good medicine.

For all the years following that incident, I have not seen the snake as a creature to be feared. The analogy, for me, has been that the snake represented the things in my life that I most feared but no longer needed to.

Nature, and the universe has my back!

CHAPTER TWENTY-SIX
The 'good old days'

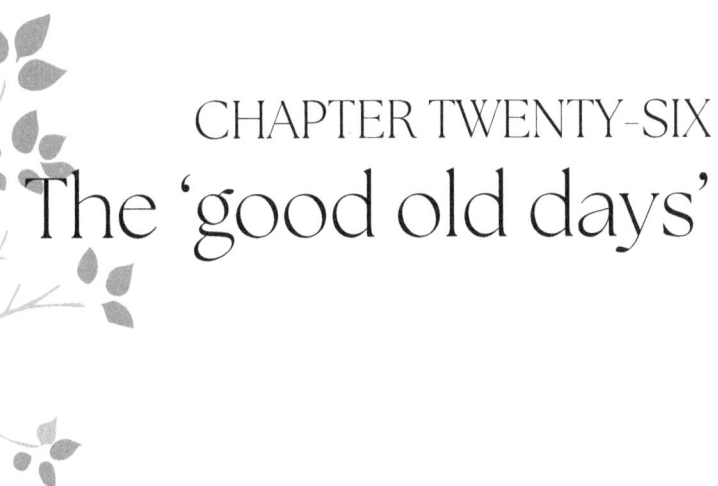

The generation of Australian baby boomers often speak with longing for the *good old days*. They were a time of more innocence – or perhaps ignorance? Childhoods, they say, were better – for some, but not for all. The stereotypical family image, beloved of advertising at the time, was white, middle class and aspirational. If you were different from that profile, life was more difficult – and always more so for First Nation people in those post-war boom years.

Moree, in north-west NSW, was a greatly divided town in the 1960s. Before the wealth that cotton brought, it was a prime wool-growing area, so there was privilege and prosperity for established landowners. The townspeople were largely homogeneous, with the only migrant family running the local café – Greek, of course. Then there were the fringe-dwelling Indigenous community, many living on missions at the edge of town, some still lived beside the riverbanks in humpies.

Our family moved to Moree when I had just commenced my first year of high school, so that my new stepfather could start his job as the Moree Shire Engineer. It was an unhappy time in our family's life, except for the joyous birth of a baby brother during a heatwave in December 1965. Babies died of dehydration during that heatwave; those of us who live first world lives forget how tough life is without the modern convenience of air-conditioning.

Our home was built up, out of the way of floodwaters, which used to inundate western river towns before levy banks were built. A wide hallway through the middle of the house acted as a breezeway, so baby Charles lived his first couple of months in a cane basket, covered with wet nappies, with a pedestal fan directed on him. At thirteen, I was our mother's willing helper, and I took great delight in the important role of keeping the nappies moist.

Early in my teen years, I gained after-school employment at a corner shop. Those corner stores were full of staple dietary goods. For those without cars and unable to walk to the main shopping centre, they were a necessity. Many of the customers were Indigenous and/or elderly. I loved my job and relished the feeling of independence my small pay packet gave me. I did question the owner one day as to why we sold Aboriginal people methylated spirits from a refrigerator. His explanation shocked me – 'I had no idea!' I still feel sickened by the toxicity of that spirit and the craving and grinding poverty that was behind the need to purchase. I couldn't work there anymore.

In 1965, the Freedom Riders, led by the activist Charles Perkins, came to Moree. I well remember that week as my stepfather, as the Shire Engineer, was embroiled in the events and I recall his distress in the evenings reporting to my mother. I believe he felt the local Indigenous people had the right to demand equal rights but wished it didn't involve the protests which impacted his work. I remember thinking it was very unfair that some of my classmates had not been allowed to attend swimming carnivals because of their skin colour. I was happy when they could do so.

The Freedom Riders highlighted the need for legislative social change at a local level, for First Nations people, who had been granted the right to vote in 1962.

In only 1962!

We really were a very White Australia back in the *good old days*.

I have no doubt my early teen experiences led me to work in Aboriginal health. It took me decades to get there, however my time in the Pilbara was the best of my nursing years and my life has been further enriched by the experiences and friendships I was afforded.

AN ETHICAL STATEMENT
'NOT THE BRUISES'

In sharing the stories of others, as well as my own, privacy and protection have been paramount. As a result, parts of some stories remain unspoken. It is a conundrum; to call out and speak of abuse in all its facets, so that it is known, or to remain silent and risk leaving everything hidden.

To not speak the entire truth, when it is not mine alone to tell, was my choice.

AUTHOR'S NOTES

One of the joys of writing this book has been in reconnecting with those of whom I have written. Seeking permission to use names and to write personal stories has developed stories within stories. In doing so I have felt determined, though nervous, to push forward to publication as I am confident there is power in sharing stories and experiences.

Friends, who were enjoying their own journey in Indigenous health in Broome, understood that I could not, in all conscience, publish any of my words without face-to-face contact and permission from my Pilbara friends and colleagues. Generously they offered me unconditional hospitality. That became three weeks of journey from Lightning Ridge to Sydney, flight to beautiful Broome, staying in their beachside home, the loan of a vehicle which enabled me to drive the 10 hours to Roebourne, revisit some of my old haunts and most importantly to spend time with those of whom I wrote. Then a bonus one week stopover in Perth spent with my friends, Kath and Stuart, and others dear to me. Treasured memories!

The collection of other permissions has not required quite so much energy however the reconnections have been heartfelt, reconfirming of friendship, trust and shared experiences. There have been lovely conversations and recalled memories.

I am most grateful that not one person has denied permission to publish after reading their "section" of the book. The two men I have been humbled by were Rick and Andrew – both ex partners have given me permission to write of them without wanting to see or know what I have written. They have simply requested a published book. I am not confident that I would have afforded them the same degree of trust however I am grateful for theirs. Love continues in a different form.

The blessing of a large extended family and a generous and varied village of friends brings me joy and is richly rewarding. It makes me rather anxious to name and thank those who have planted the seed of thought and encouraged me to find the confidence to write the stories. There may be others that I risk offending!

My sister-in-law Beth, a registered nurse, has quietly planted seeds of professional encouragement for some years. A friend Judy, who comes from a life of privilege, took the time to ring me one day and tell me that my life story was courageous and should be written. Andrew's sister Josephine, a published poet, read a story I wrote and told me not to lose my voice. A girl I met on the first day of our nursing training, Denise, has been a lifelong friend. We have always lived a long distance apart and used to stay in touch by letter during the years that we worked and raised our families. Denise has been the final nail – the just do it!!

It was to Denise that I sent the first draft of my words as I trusted her as an avid reader, professional nurse and friend. Denise was kind and encouraging but insisted I could dive down and tell more. My daughters, Rebel and Deanne, read the first final edit and said, "get messy", to tell more of my story. I have got as "messy" as I am comfortable with and I am so very grateful to those three women for challenging me to share more of my personal story.

FINAL WORD

Rather than be overwhelmed by the need, in my chosen profession, I have always been strengthened by the Star Thrower story by Loren Eiseley. There are different versions retold and adapted since the late 1960s, but in my words:

"A young boy stands on a beach littered by thousands of stranded, dying starfish. He is methodically bending, picking up and throwing back into the sea one starfish after another. A man walking along sneers at him and says, 'You will never make a difference.' The boy bends, picks up another starfish and throws it into the sea and says to the man, 'I made a difference to that one.'"

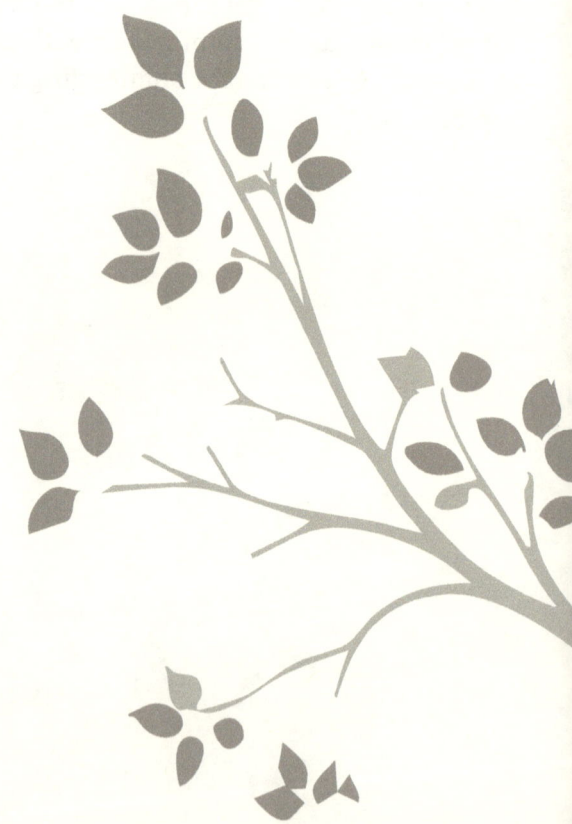

ACKNOWLEDGEMENTS

I wish to acknowledge that Australia, the country on which I was blessed to be born, to have worked, travelled and loved, was never ceded.

I pay my respects to all who have gone before me and acknowledge the First Nation elder's past, present and emerging who hold the ancient stories and culture of this glorious land.

Heartfelt thanks to Dr Michael Bartram, Ruth Ni Scanlain Hackett and Natahsa Gilmour who took the time in their busy professional lives to read my words and to find their own for testimonials. You gave me courage to move forward in publication and I thank you.

My sincere thanks to Jacqueline Gaul, Author, who introduced me to my editor, Natasha Gilmour, Kind Press. My fledging book and confidence as a first-time author could not have been placed in more thoughtful care. Then Jacqui Webster, Author, who introduced me to Jessica Mudditt, Author, Publisher and founder Hembury Books. I live in some isolation with no connection to the world of writing and publishing, so all these introductions come with stories of serendipity, connection and conversation. Then, when I desperately needed someone to re edit three chapters I had added to, close to publication, a cottage guest asked me if I was a writer, Tricia Fitzgerald, Kirby Communications, was an editor.

I thank the Hembury Books team. I am not going to name you all as, at the time of writing, there are a couple of months to go before the launch of Not Just a Nurse. The professional and personal care of Jessica and Grace, to date, assures me that the presentation of my words is in very good hands and I am so very grateful.

So many people have played a role in the evolution of my memoir. I am privileged by the friends and family who have listened, advised and supported.

BOOKS MENTIONED

Fraser, T 1992, *For better, for worse and for lunch*, HarperCollins, Sydney.

Flannery, T 1994, *The future eaters*, Reed Books, Port Melbourne.

Lee, T 2006, *Lonesome for my country*, Magabala Books, Broome.

Mahood, K 2022, *Wandering with intent: essays*, Scribe Publications, Melbourne.

Porter, EH 1913, *Pollyanna*, L.C. Page & Co., Boston.

Rees, P 2008, *The ANZAC girls*, Allen & Unwin, Sydney.

Shoffstall, VA n.d., *After a while*, poem, various online and print editions.

www.ingramcontent.com/pod-product-compliance
Lightning Source LLC
Chambersburg PA
CBHW060458080526
44584CB00015B/1468